Meeting the Challenges of Oral and Head and Neck Cancer

A SURVIVOR'S GUIDE

D1057565

Meeting the Challenges of Oral and Head and Neck Cancer

A SURVIVOR'S GUIDE

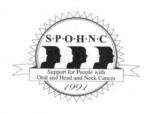

Edited by
Nancy E. Leupold, MA
James J. Sciubba, DMD, PhD

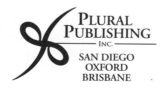

PLURAL
PUBLISHING
INC.
SAN DIEGO
OXFORD
BRISBANE

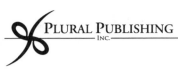

PLURAL PUBLISHING
INC.

5521 Ruffin Road
San Diego, CA 92123

e-mail: info@pluralpublishing.com
Web site: http://www.pluralpublishing.com

49 Bath Street
Abingdon, Oxfordshire OX14 1EA
United Kingdom

Copyright © by Plural Publishing, Inc. 2008

Typeset in 11/13 Garamond Book by Flanagan's Publishing Services, Inc.
Printed in the United States of America by McNaughton & Gunn, Inc.

All rights, including that of translation, reserved. No part of this publication may
be reproduced, stored in a retrieval system, or transmitted in any form or by any
means, electronic, mechanical, recording, or otherwise, including photocopying,
recording, taping, Web distribution, or information storage and retrieval systems
without the prior written consent of the publisher.

For permission to use material from this text, contact us by
Telephone: (866) 758-7251
Fax: (888) 758-7255
e-mail: permissions@pluralpublishing.com

*Every attempt has been made to contact the copyright holders for material
originally printed in another source. If any have been inadvertently overlooked,
the publishers will gladly make the necessary arrangements at the first
opportunity.*

Cover Design by René Rodriguez, Rhino Graphica LLC

Library of Congress Cataloging-in-Publication Data:

Meeting the challenges of oral and head and neck cancer : a survivor's guide /
[edited by] Nancy E. Leupold and James J. Sciubba.
     p. ; cm.
  Includes bibliographical references and index.
  ISBN-13: 978-1-59756-239-3 (alk. paper)
  ISBN-10: 1-59756-239-4 (alk. paper)
  1. Head–Cancer–Patients–Rehabilitation. 2. Neck–Cancer–Patients–Rehabilitation.
  [DNLM: 1. Head and Neck Neoplasms–therapy. 2. Continuity of Patient Care.
3. Head and Neck Neoplasms–complications. 4. Head and Neck Neoplasms–
psychology. 5. Physician-Patient Relations. 6. Survivors. WE 707 C437 2007]
I. Leupold, Nancy E. II. Sciubba, James J.
  RC280.H4C43 2007
  616.99'491–dc22

                                                                2007045748

CONTENTS

v

FOREWORD

Survivors of head and neck cancer should welcome this volume, which, as its title suggests, is a guide to assist in recognizing, alleviating, and solving problems that can accompany cancer of the head and neck and its treatment. The contributors include survivors, caregivers, and health care providers, including surgeons, radiation and medical oncologists, dentists and maxillofacial prosthodontists, speech and swallowing therapists, dietitians, social workers, dermatologists, and nurses. The multiplicity of contributors is a reflection of the complexity of the treatment and the myriad of complications and consequences that accompany the treatment of head and neck cancer. Head and neck cancer includes tumors that may involve one or several individual anatomic sites within the head and neck region. These comprise a complex and varied group of neoplasms with somewhat unpredictable natural history and varying response to treatment and that have varying effects upon the patient, depending upon the site of origin, size, and extent of the tumor. Generalizations often do not apply to specific patients and their specific tumors.

Treatment may vary widely and must be properly selected and administered to most appropriately treat both the patient and the tumor. One or more of the previously mentioned health care providers may be involved in the adequate and complete care and rehabilitation of the patient with head and neck cancer. It is important that the patient have access to any and all of these disciplines/therapists to ensure that adequate and complete treatment and care are available. What that treatment may include is a vital matter to be decided at the outset, subject to change as necessary as time and treatment proceed and hopefully directed by a knowledgeable, experienced, and conscientious physician/surgeon. It is most important that the physician thoroughly discusses with the patient and responsible family members the treatment options; the potential complications and side effects, both early and late; and the antici- pated results. Good communication between doctor/therapist and patient is mandatory and hopefully will begin with the initial encounter and continue throughout the treatment, recovery, reha- bilitation, and the long-term follow-up. It is also apparent that one of these doctors should be the team leader, the "captain of the ship," overseeing both the multiple caregivers and monitoring the patient's treatment and clinical course. It is this leader to whom the patient and family can look for guidance, information, direction, encour- agement, and reassurance.

As is well documented in this volume, the treatment of head and neck cancer can be complex; time consuming; morbid; and beset with complications and side effects that will adversely affect the patient's function, appearance, and quality of life. With careful initial patient evaluation, proper planning, close observation, and follow-up during treatment and beyond, some side effects may be minimized, if not prevented, and all side effects may be treated early and more effectively.

The goal of *Meeting the Challenges of Oral and Head and Neck Cancer: A Survivor's Guide* is to educate the patient about the numerous and varied side effects of treatment and to guide the patient in their recognition and treatment. The importance of this recognition cannot be overemphasized because such complica- tions may be life threatening at worst, or interfere with the proper continuity of treatment or stimulate intermediate and long-term consequences at the least. Careful and continuous follow-up, obser- vation, and examination of the patient during and following treat- ment are imperative. Such follow-up may continue for the remainder of the patient's life, so the quality of the doctor-patient relationship is vitally important. Treatment may need to be altered or temporarily interrupted depending upon the clinical course. Close communica- tion between patients and their therapist/caregivers is imperative so that the professionals are fully aware of the patient's status at all times. It is the patient's responsibility to recognize and report adverse symptoms early on to the responsible medical personnel so that appropriate corrective or palliative measures and treatment can be promptly initiated. It should also be noted that the physician in charge is the individual to whom vital questions and observations should be directed, not to relatives, fellow patients, or technicians.

Each chapter of this book addresses a specific aspect of head and neck cancer, from the introduction in Chapter 1 through discussions of challenges of various treatments, challenges of responses to treatment on various anatomic sites and functions, challenges of economic and insurance issues, discussions of clinical trials, and enumeration of treatment products and therapies and informative literature. Any directed therapy should be discussed with, and approved by, the responsible medical provider, either surgeon, radiation oncologist, or medical oncologist. The Internet can be a source of information; however, it should be noted that the information obtained may not always be correct or appropriate for the individual patient and his or her clinical situation. Treatment *must* be individualized to best fit the patient and his or her response to such treatment.

The editors and contributors to this volume are to be congratulated for compiling a source of information and practical advice not heretofore available. With the benefit of this information and advice, and under the guidance of the responsible physician(s), hopefully the course of the treatment of the patient with head and neck cancer will be optimized, individualized, and modified to ensure the maximum therapeutic benefit to the patient while preserving optimal quality of life.

Elliot W. Strong, MD, FACS
Emeritus, Memorial Hospital for Cancer and Allied
    Disease
Emeritus, Memorial Sloan-Kettering Cancer Center
Former Attending Surgeon and Chief, Head and
    Neck Service
Former Professor of Surgery at Cornell University
    Medical College

PREFACE

Head and neck cancers comprise a variety of malignant tumors that may occur in the head and neck region, namely the oral cavity, the pharynx (throat), the cervical esophagus, the paranasal sinuses and nasal cavity, the larynx, and the thyroid and the salivary glands. Lesions of the facial skin, scalp, and neck and the cervical lymph nodes may also be classified as head and neck cancers.

Although the prevalence of oral and head and neck cancer in the United States is only about 3 to 4% of all cancers diagnosed, the importance of these diseases is heightened by the fact that functional problems and esthetic differences are commonly associated with this type of cancer and its treatment. Indeed, coping with oral and head and neck cancer can be extremely difficult. Not only is a person dealing with a diagnosis that can be life-threatening, but he or she must also deal with possible alterations in facial appearance, speech, and the senses of smell and taste, swallowing, and vision. These alterations, in turn, may lead to considerable threats to one's self-image, confidence, identity, and emotional balance. No body part is so exposed to the world as a person's face, head, and neck. Other scars and deformities of the body may be covered, but it is difficult to hide disfigurements and treatment-associated dysfunctions of the oral cavity and head and neck.

As a result of the ongoing changes in the treatment of oral and head and neck cancer and the use of the Internet to obtain information, patients and their families are becoming increasingly more active in researching and identifying their options for care. The capability of patients to more actively participate in their own care has increased the need for education and awareness of the various and often overwhelming information that is available through the Internet. This level of patient empowerment has begun to change the doctor-patient relationship with the patient and family being more involved than ever in treatment decisions and understanding the levels of risk and anticipated benefits of proposed treatment.

Since the founding of Support for People with Oral and Head and Neck Cancer (SPOHNC) in 1991, we have had the opportunity to speak with thousands of survivors who have undergone various treatments for their cancers. Most discover that there are only limited and reliable resources available to them concerning head and neck cancer. This, in turn, has led to patients and their families to contact SPOHNC for help in finding answers to specific questions related to their individual cancer journeys in thoughtful and patient-directed ways.

Meeting the Challenges of Oral and Head and Neck Cancer: A Survivors Guide offers the patient, caregiver, family, and friends the opportunity to learn about a difficult cancer and its associated treatment options as well as some of the psychosocial aspects of living with the disease and its aftermath. Information concerning dental care, skin care, communication and swallowing difficulties, nutrition, insurance issues, and clinical trials is also included in this book which provides numerous resources in each chapter or section. *Meeting the Challenges of Oral and Head and Neck Cancer: A Survivors Guide*, uses a novel approach in Chapter 11, where tables of products, therapies, and survivor input provide information and supportive care to head and neck cancer survivors facing the challenges of side effects or lingering effects of treatment.

Meeting the Challenges of Oral and Head and Neck Cancer: A Survivors Guide is one of very few books written in user-friendly, patient-directed language about oral and head and neck cancer. With all that this book encompasses, it is a "must-have" reference for survivors, caregivers, family, and friends as well as health care professionals involved in the management of oral and head and neck cancer patients.

Nancy E. Leupold, M.A.
Survivor, President and Founder
SPOHNC

James J. Sciubba, D.M.D., Ph.D
Vice President and Chairman, Medical Advisory Board
SPOHNC

ACKNOWLEDGMENTS

SPOHNC is most grateful to the many authors who supported this book with their contributions of chapters and sections providing information for oral and head and neck cancer survivors and their caregivers and to Monica Pfister for her help in revising language in Chapter 3 to make it more suitable for the lay reader.

Many survivors, family members, and health care professionals also offered suggestions and input for the resource tables in this book. We greatly appreciate the contributions of John Acton, Trisha Appelhans. Sandra Ashley, Sandy Bates, Charlie Bauer, Joseph R. Bauer, Janis Beard, Michael Birnbaum, Lawrie Bloom, Marie Boland, Patricia M. Boldt, Mary Grace Bontempo, Stephen Bortz, Boston SPOHNC Chapter, Richard Boucher, Addie Brown, Sheryl Bunton, Rita Burfitt, Emily and Dennis Carroll, Kathleen A. Castillo, John M. Chambers, Kathy Chambers, Barry Cooper, Lillian Corbett, Gene Covington, Joan Cummings, David Curbello, Dallas SPOHNC Chapter, Allison Dekker, RN, Hank V. Deneski, Bette L. Denlinger, Sal and Jean Diana, John P. Dowling, Gail Fass, Evelyn Fowler, Peach Gazda, Vince Gilhool, Karyl L. Gill, Carol Glavin, Mike Golub, Lynn Gormley, John Groves, Elizabeth Hadas, Marilyn Haines, Gabriel Hamilton, Michael Henault, Dave Hepburn, Jerry Hepburn, Pam Hoff, Henry V. Holdridge, Carol Humphries, Jack Igleburger, Indianapolis South SPOHNC Chapter, Neal Isaacs, Kansas City SPOHNC Chapter, Dianne Kiyomoto-Kuey, RD, Robert R. Klauber, Lee Laino, Jeffrey Langdale, Leonard Lanyo, Pat Laumann, Janice Leak, Linda Legendre, Danny Lindburg, Ann Linkh, Los Angeles-UCLA SPOHNC Chapter, Robin Luo, Gail B. Mackiernan, Carolyn Martocchia, Joe Meditz, Larry Menkoff, Martha Miller, Thomas E. Momeyer, Dwayne and Barbara Moore, Micki Naimoli, Lisa and Tuan Nguyen, NJ-Philadelphia SPOHNC Chapter, Bill Parisi, Pat and Felix Quinn, Phil E. and Naomi Reimer, Sharon A. Renkes, Sanford Riesenfeld, Jerome P. Rothstein, DDS,

MHA, Jerry Runyon, Ernst Schneck, E.J. Scott, Joann Scott, Bob Simpson, Sandra L. Smith, Dan Stack, Dennis Staropoli, Alice Steiner, Nancy Symonds, RDH, Valerie Doreen Targia, Sharon Tupa, George Tyson, Chuck Van Alen, Janet Wallstadt, Madelyn Walsh, Mark H. Weiss, Bill and Ann Wesp, Sheila West, Allen Wilson, Mary Ellyn Witt, RN, Jan Wundsam, Tom Yohe, and the many others who through the years have shared their stories and provided support and encouragement to others.

Meeting the Challenges of Oral and Head and Neck Cancer: A Survivor's Guide began as an idea for bringing practical information to oral and head and neck cancer survivors and their caregivers in a reader-friendly format. We would like to express our sincere appreciation to SPOHNC's board of directors and its medical advisory board and to Amgen Oncology for their interest in this idea and for their support of this new type of book that we hope will be of help to many.

And for the research and dedication in helping to provide information for the tables and resources, we gratefully acknowledge the work of SPOHNC staff members Janine Cortese and Mary Ann Caputo.

Thank you so very much, one and all.

CONTRIBUTORS

Julie Blair, MA, CCC-SLP
Clinical Instructor
MUSC Evelyn Trammell Institute
for Voice and Swallowing
Adjunct Faculty
College of Health Professions
Medical University of South
Carolina
Charleston, SC
Chapter 7

David M. Brizel, MD
Professor of Radiation Oncology
Associate Professor of
Otolaryngology Head and Neck
Surgery
Duke Comprehensive Cancer Center
Duke University Medical Center
Durham, NC
Chapter 3

Beth Darnley
Chief Program Officer
Patient Advocate Foundation
Newport News, VA
Chapter 9A

Scott E. Davis, Esq.
Disability Attorney
Phoenix, AZ
Chapter 9C

Patty Delaney
Director

Cancer Liaison Program
Food and Drug Administration
Office of Special Health Issues
Rockville, MD
Chapter 10B

Gail Funk, RN, OCN
Clinical Nurse IV
Department of Radiation
Oncology
Duke University Hospital System
Durham, NC
Chapter 3

Matthew G. Fury, MD, PhD
Assistant Attending Physician
Memorial Sloan-Kettering Cancer
Center
New York, NY
Chapter 4

Mary Giguere, RN, BSN
Director, Colorectal CareLine
Patient Advocate Foundation
Newport News, VA
Chapter 9A

Linda Gilliard, MS, RD, CNSD
Clinical Dietitian
Radiation Oncology Clinic
Duke University Medical Center
Durham, NC
Chapter 3

Constance L. Goodman, RN
Patient Services Administrator
Patient Advocate Foundation
Newport News, VA
Chapter 9A

Malinda Heuring
Director of Education
National Foundation for
    Ectodermal Dysplasias (NFED)
Mascoutah, IL
Chapter 9B

Mario E. Lacouture, MD
Assistant Professor
Director, Cancer Skin Care Program
Department of Dermatology
Robert H Lurie Comprehensive
    Cancer Center
Northwestern University
Chicago, IL
Chapter 6

Nancy E. Leupold, MA
Survivor, President and Founder
Support for People with Oral and
    Head and Neck Cancer
    (SPOHNC)
Locust Valley, NY
Chapters 10A and 11

Tami Lewis RN, CCM
Senior Clinical Case Manager
Patient Advocate Foundation
Newport News, VA
Chapter 9A

Su Hsien Lim, MD
Head and Neck Medical Oncology
    Fellow
Memorial Sloan-Kettering Cancer
    Center
New York, NY
Chapter 4

**Bonnie Martin-Harris, PhD,
CCC-SLP, BRS-S**
Director, MUSC Evelyn Trammell
    Institute for Voice and
    Swallowing
Associate Professor,
    Otolaryngology—Head and
    Neck Surgery
Medical University of South
    Carolina
Charleston, SC
Chapter 7

**Eugene N. Myers, MD, FACS,
FRCS Edin. (Hon)**
Distinguished Professor and
    Emeritus Chair
Department of Otolaryngology
University of Pittsburgh School
    of Medicine and Medical
    Center
Pittsburgh, PA
Chapter 2

David Myssiorek, MD, FACS
Professor of Otolaryngology
New York University School of
    Medicine
New York, NY
Chapter 1

David G. Pfister, MD
Chief, Head and Neck Medical
    Oncology Service
Co-leader, Head and Neck Cancer
    Disease Management Team
Memorial Sloan-Kettering Cancer
    Center
Professor of Medicine
Weill Medical College of Cornell
    University
New York, NY
Chapter 4

Mary Kaye Richter
Executive Director and Founder
National Foundation for
    Ectodermal Dysplasias (NFED)
Mascoutah, IL
Chapter 9B

Mary Ann Downey Rubio
Senior PA-C
Department of Radiation Oncology
Duke University Medical Center
Durham, NC
Chapter 3

James J. Sciubba, DMD, PhD
The Milton J. Dance Head & Neck
    Cancer Center
The Greater Baltimore Medical
    Center
Baltimore, MD
Professor, Ret., The Johns Hopkins
    Medical School
Department of Otolaryngology,
    Head and Neck Surgery
Chapter 5

Connie Slayton, BSN
Program Director, CDC/PAF Center
Prevention and Survivorship
    Partnership
Patient Advocate Foundation
Newport News, VA
Chapter 9A

**Jennifer Thompson, RD, LD,
CNSD**
Senior Clinical Dietitian
Department of Oncology and
    Blood and Marrow Transplant
Baylor University Medical Center
Dallas, TX
Chapter 8

Tanya Walker, RN, BSN
Senior Clinical Case Manager
Patient Advocate Foundation
Newport News, VA
Chapter 9A

Dedicated to the memory of
David P. Wolk, MD, FACS,
a kind and gentle man and a
compassionate head and neck surgeon
whose support and encouragement
led to the founding of
Support for People with Oral and Head and Neck Cancer
(SPOHNC)

1

INTRODUCTION TO THE CHALLENGES OF ORAL AND HEAD AND NECK CANCER

David Myssiorek, MD, FACS

Head and neck cancer (HNC) encompasses a group of tumors that arise from the structures of the upper aerodigestive tract. Classically, these include all of the structures that are involved with swallowing, speaking, and breathing (mouth, throat, nose, sinuses, larynx, and upper esophagus); salivary glands (parotid gland, submandibular gland, sublingual gland, and minor salivary glands); thyroid gland and parathyroid glands; and the ear and skin of the head and neck. Additionally, the lymph nodes of the neck are always considered when dealing with cancers of these organs.

Diverse tumors, both benign and malignant, can arise from these structures. Many different salivary gland tumors and thyroid tumors are found yearly, but the most common cancer of the head and neck in adults is squamous cell carcinoma. Squamous cell carcinoma arises from the cells that line the upper aerodigestive tract, sinuses, and skin. This resource book will address the treatments and their aftereffects for people with head and neck cancer.

Anatomy

The subsites of the upper aerodigestive tract include the mouth, nose, sinuses, pharynx, larynx, and neck. The oral cavity starts at the exposed margins of the upper and lower lips called the vermilion border. Because of a rich vascular supply to the lip and a thin covering, the vermilion appears redder than skin. The mucous membrane covering the cheeks and lips running from the upper gum to the lower gum lines is known as the buccal mucosa. A triangular area extending medially (inward) to the region between the buccal mucosa and the space between the upper and lower gum is called the retromolar trigone. The oral cavity ends at the junction of the hard and soft palates.

The tongue is divided into thirds. The front two thirds of the tongue is considered a structure of the oral cavity and is responsible for speech/articulation and helps to move food to the teeth for chewing and backward for swallowing. The undersurface of the tongue (ventral tongue) blends into the floor of the mouth. The floor of the mouth is located between the dental-bearing tissues of

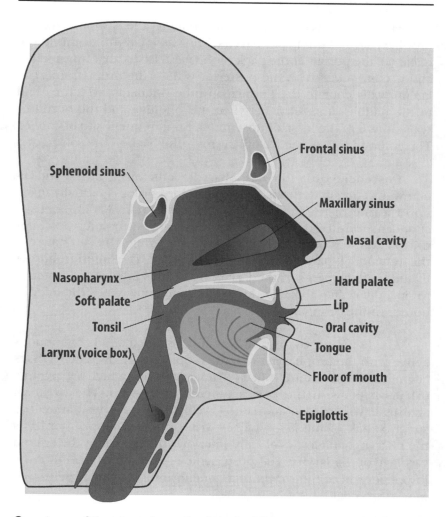

Courtesy of the American Society for Therapeutic Radiology and Oncology (ASTRO)

the lower jaw and bears the ducts of both submandibular glands. The alveolar ridge is the structure that contains the teeth and gums. There is a lower (mandibular) alveolus and upper (maxillary) alveolus. The hard palate marks the posterior extent of the oral cavity. To a degree, oral cavity structures develop from embryological structures arising from the cranial nerve associated with mastication (chewing).

The pharynx is divided into three regions: the nasopharynx, the oropharynx, and the hypopharynx. The nasopharynx begins at the choanae, the portals at the back of the nasal cavity that transmit air, and is continuous with the posterior wall of the oropharynx. The lateral walls contain the Eustachian tube openings, which extend to the middle ear. A cleft between this opening and the posterior wall known as the fossa of Rosenmüller is a frequent site of cancer. The anterior wall of the nasopharynx is the back of the soft palate.

Descending from the nasopharynx is the oropharynx. The lateral walls contain the tonsils. The anterior border is partially made up of a ring of tissue known as Waldeyer's ring, which contains abundant tonsillar-type tissue. The base of the tongue (posterior third) and the tonsils are part of Waldeyer's ring. The soft palate is the remaining part of the anterior border. The inferior border includes attachments to the larynx by various folds and ligaments. An imaginary line through the hyoid bone demarcates the inferior border of the oropharynx.

The hypopharynx is roughly funnel shaped and is continuous above with the oropharynx and the esophagus below. The recesses lateral to the larynx are called pyriform sinuses, which are pyramidal in shape with the apices pointed downward. The pyriform sinuses have a medial and lateral wall. The medial wall abuts the superior half of the larynx. The pyriform sinus's upper border is the pharyngoepiglottic fold and inferiorly the apex is at the cricoid cartilage of the larynx. The postcricoid area is the back end of the lower portion of the larynx that contains most of the muscles that move the vocal folds.

The larynx forms at the end of the trachea and "buds" into the pharynx during embryogenesis. The larynx is made of bone, cartilage, and muscle. It is divided into a superior or upper half, which is mostly sensory (allowing perception of food/liquid before it enters the windpipe). There is little motor function. The epiglottis acts as a keel to divert food and liquid to the sides away from the laryngeal opening. The inferior or lower half contains the motor parts of the larynx—the vocal folds. The space between them is the glottis. The vocal folds form a complex valve that allows us to hold our breath and block matter from entering the lungs. When damaged or paralyzed, aspiration can occur. Secondarily, the vocal folds are responsible for voice. The vocal folds are attached to the thyroid cartilage anteriorly and to the arytenoid cartilages posteriorly. The arytenoid cartilages can move side to side and front to back and thus are capable of moving the vocal folds in complex ways, creating the human larynx's range of sounds. All of the muscles that attach to the arytenoids are innervated by the recurrent laryngeal nerve, which is a major branch of the vagus nerve.

Incidence

The incidence of HNC has stabilized. In 2007, 34,360 new cases of cancer of the oral cavity and pharynx are expected, approximately one third in the tongue, one third in the mouth, and one third in the throat (Jemal et al., 2007). Another 11,300 cases are predicted in the larynx and 33,500 cases in the thyroid. Comparatively, during this same year, 213,380 lung cancers, 218,890 prostate cancers, and 178,480 breast cancers are estimated.

Oral cavity and pharynx cancers account for 3% of all cancers in men and less than 1% in women. From 1991 to 2003, the death rate for these tumors decreased from 2.03 per 100,000 women to 1.47 per 100,000 women, representing an overall change of 27% in women. Similarly, men have experienced a drop from 5.61 per 100,000 to 4.06 per 100,000, representing an overall change of 27%. In men, death from laryngeal cancer has also decreased. There has been an improvement in the 5-year survival rate for the oral cavity (all stages included) from 53% in 1975 to 60% in 2002 (Jemal et al., 2007).

Etiology

Risk factors for the development of head and neck cancer include tobacco use (smoking, chewing, and snuff forms of smokeless tobacco) and reverse smoking (Decker & Goldstein, 1982), which is smoking with the lighted end inside the mouth; alcohol consumption (Strome et al., 2002); betel nut/paan chewing; and sun exposure of the lips and skin. Other suspected etiologies include human papillomavirus (Licitra et al., 2006; Snijders et al., 1992; D'Souza et al., 2007), reflux disease (Qadeer, Colabianchi, Strome, & Vaezi, 2006; Locke, Talley, & Fett, 1999), and a familial predisposition (Copper et al., 1995). Some evidence exists that some laryngeal cancers may be related to occupational risks (Brown et al., 1988; Flanders & Rothman, 1982).

Squamous cell cancer represents more than 95% of all cancers of the upper aerodigestive tract. It is commonly associated with smoking and/or alcohol abuse. It is estimated that a person who smokes has 15 to 20 times the risk for developing head and neck cancer whereas alcohol abuse carries 2 to 3 times the risk for HNC. P53 is a tumor suppressor gene whose mutation is associated with the development of upper aerodigestive tract cancer. These genetic mutations increase with smoking and drinking. Ninety-five percent of HNC is found in smokers. In Southeast Asia the practice of wrapping betel in paan and chewing the product has been linked to oral cavity cancers. In Bombay approximately 50% of head and neck cancers are buccal cancers related to this practice. Chewing paan increases the risk of developing HNC by 2.8 times, and this number rises dramatically when chewing paan is combined with smoking.

Human papillomavirus (HPV) types 16 and 18 have been found in laryngeal verrucous cancers and tongue and tonsil cancers. In a study from the Mayo Clinic (Strome et al., 2002), 46% of tonsil cancers examined had HPV DNA identified in the cancer cells. Only 6% of normal tonsils had HPV DNA copies. Most recently, studies have been published that have confirmed this relationship in which the specific etiology of oropharyngeal squamous carcinoma was strongly linked with oral HPV infection with or without the known associated risk factors of tobacco use and alcohol consumption (D'Souza et al., 2007).

Nasopharyngeal cancer is the most common cancer in China and is associated with a rise in the titre of anti-Epstein-Barr viral capsid antigens antibodies. The risk of people in Kwang Tung Province developing nasopharyngeal cancer is 25 times that of a Caucasian population. When people migrate from Kwang Tung, the increased risk of cancer persists but is decreased.

Some authors believe that some laryngeal cancers may be linked to laryngopharyngeal reflux (LPR) (Qadeer et al., 2006; Locke et al., 1999). The evidence supporting a direct cause and effect of LPR and laryngeal cancer is lacking at this time (Qadeer et al., 2006). Many earlier studies were poorly controlled. LPR has been found in approximately 40% of the U.S. population. Both smoking and alcohol consumption increase the likelihood of reflux (Locke et al., 1999). It is extremely difficult to isolate LPR as a cause of cancer.

Sun exposure is a known cause of both melanoma and non-melanomatous skin cancers. The lips are particularly prone to squamous cell cancer from sun exposure.

Squamous Cell Carcinoma

Several types of cancers affect the lining of the upper aerodigestive tract. Besides squamous cell cancer, minor salivary gland cancers, adenocarcinomas, and metastases from other cancers involve the head and neck. Squamous cell cancer is graded by the level of cellular differentiation. Well-differentiated cancers resemble the original cell from which they arose. The squamous cell is designed to line our mouths and throats, our sinuses, and all of our skin. It is a "wear and tear" lining and is waterproof. It produces keratin, which can readily be found in cuticles, nails, and hands and feet. Cancer of this cell occurs when its DNA is altered and the cell proliferates in an independent or ungoverned fashion. Well-differentiated cancers tend to behave better than poorly differentiated cancers. The less differentiated a cell is, the less like the cell of origin it appears and the more invasive it becomes. The differentiation of the cancerous cell does not affect staging and is not often a predictor of outcome.

Variants of squamous cell carcinoma reflect special differentiation such as spindle cell or glandular differentiation. One variant, papillary carcinoma, behaves differently at the micro- and macroscopic level. Verrucous carcinoma closely resembles a wart, is slow growing, and rarely metastasizes but is locally destructive and is frequently mistaken for more benign tumors. Generally, however, squamous cell cancer and its variants behave similarly and are treated similarly.

Squamous cell cancer starts as a clone of cells that reside within the epithelium or lining and proliferates within this layer initially. When limited to this epithelium, the entity is known as carcinoma in situ or CIS. If these cells invade through the basement membrane (a layer of collagen and glycoproteins that supports the epithelium and separates it from the underlying connective tissue), it is considered to be invasive and gains the potential to spread to regional lymph nodes in the neck and beyond.

Two terms require explanation. *Leukoplakia* is any white patch on a mucous membrane that doesn't wipe off. It usually indicates a state of damage or tissue alteration. It does not necessarily mean cancer since irritation by devices such as dentures and local trauma can result in leukoplakia. *Erythroplakia* is a velvety red lesion found on mucous membranes. This is usually more sinister than leukoplakia and requires investigation by biopsy.

A major concept in modern diagnosis and treatment is that of field cancerization (Slaughter, Southwick, & Smejkal, 1953). Simply put, whatever allowed one cell to differentiate to a cancer (environment, irritants, radiation, genetics) can readily induce the same effect in other cells. This is why some patients develop multiple cancers within the upper aerodigestive tract. It is estimated that 20% of head and neck cancer patients will develop a second cancer. During the evaluation of a patient with head and neck cancer, physicians may order imaging studies and perform *panendoscopy* (a combination of laryngoscopy, esophagoscopy, and bronchoscopy) to seek out these second primary cancers.

Treatment Modalities

Treatment of head and neck cancer must take several factors into consideration. The age and health of the patient frequently determine how aggressive treatment can be. Some patients with liver disease from alcohol use often cannot tolerate certain chemotherapy regimens. The older patient with significant heart disease and other forms of medical compromise may not be able to tolerate a very lengthy cancer operation and reconstruction. Patients who have already had radiation therapy usually cannot get additional radiation therapy to the same area. Patients with Fanconi's anemia frequently have adverse reactions to radiation therapy, making it difficult to deliver such treatment safely (Bagby & Alter, 2006). The size of the lesion helps determine the stage of the disease, which in turn will affect most treatment plans. Patients with metastases to the neck require more therapy, usually a combination of treatment modalities. Distant metastases (lung, liver, bone, and brain) usually portend a poor outcome, and major surgical procedures are not undertaken in this situation with unusual exceptions.

Treatment is determined by a multidisciplinary team in most locations in the United States. Tumor boards serve in an advisory fashion and consist of otolaryngologists, head and neck surgeons, plastic and reconstructive surgeons, radiation oncologists, medical oncologists, oral surgeons, pathologists, prosthodontists, nurses, speech language pathologists, social workers, residents, and students. Early lesions (stage I and II) can usually be treated effectively by either radiation therapy or surgery. Later stage lesions (stage III and IV) usually require at least two treatment modalities, that is, radiation therapy and surgery or radiation therapy and chemotherapy. Many methods are used to determine the extent of disease prior to treatment planning. CT scan, MRIs, nuclear medical scans, endoscopy and biopsy, physical examination, and analysis of patient symptoms all figure into the evaluation of the cancer and hence the treatment plan.

Head and neck cancers and their treatment differ from other human cancers in several ways. Because the majority of head and neck cancers are tobacco and/or alcohol related, it is clear that most of these cancers are preventable. The structures of the head and neck are necessary for breathing, speaking, eating, hearing, seeing, smelling, and tasting. We contact our environment mainly through the head and neck. Cancers of this region and their treatment may result in deficits of any of these structures and their corresponding function. The person with oral and head and neck cancer requires greater rehabilitation, emotional support, and quality of life improvement than patients with most other cancers. In recent years, strides have been made to emphasize the important roles of prevention, early detection and treatment, and reconstruction of head and neck cancer defects. These efforts have resulted in decreasing numbers of many forms of head and neck cancer, improved quality of life, and improved survival rates.

References

Bagby, G. C., & Alter, B. P. (2006). Fanconi anemia. *Seminars in Hematology*, *43*, 147-156.

Brown, L. M., Mason, T. J., Pickle, L. W., Stewart, P. A., Buffler, P. A., Burau, K., et al. (1988). Occupational risk factors for laryngeal cancer on the Texas Gulf Coast. *Cancer Research*, *48*, 1960-1964.

Copper, M. P., Jovanovic, A., Nauta, J. J., Braakhuis, B. J., de Vries, N., van der Waal, I., et al. (1995). Role of genetic factors in the etiology of squamous cell carcinoma of the head and neck. *Archives of Otolaryngology—Head and Neck Surgery*, *121*, 157-160.

Decker, J., & Goldstein, J. C. (1982). Risk factors in head and neck cancer. *New England Journal of Medicine*, *306*, 1151-1155.

D'Souza, G., Kreimer, A. R., Viscidi, M., Pawlita, M., Fahkry, C., Koch, W. M., et al. (2007). Case-control study of human papillomavirus and oropharyngeal cancer. *New England Journal of Medicine*, *356*, 1944-1956.

Flanders, W. D., & Rothman, K. J. (1982). Occupational risk for laryngeal cancer. *American Journal of Public Health*, *72*, 369-372.

Jemal, A., Siegel, R., Ward, E., Murray, T., Xu, J., & Thun, M. J. (2007). Cancer statistics, 2007. *CA: A Cancer Journal for Clinicians*, *57*, 43-66.

Licitra, L., Perrone, F., Bossi, P., Suardi, S., Mariani, L., Artusi, R., et al. (2006). High-risk human papillomavirus affects prognosis in patients with surgically treated oropharyngeal squamous cell carcinoma. *Journal of Clinical Oncology*, *24*, 5630-5636.

Locke, G. R., III, Talley, N. J., & Fett, S. L. (1999). Risk factors associated with symptoms of gastroesophageal reflux. *American Journal of Medicine*, *106*, 642-649.

Qadeer, M. A., Colabianchi, N., Strome, M., & Vaezi, M. F. (2006). Gastroesophageal reflux and laryngeal cancer: Causation or association? A critical review. *American Journal of Otolaryngology*, *27*, 119-128.

Slaughter, D. P., Southwick, H. W., & Smejkal, W. (1953). "Field cancerization" in oral stratified squamous epithelium. *Cancer*, *6*, 963-968.

Snijders, P. J., Cromme, F. V., van den Brule, A. J., Schrijnemakers, H. F., Snow, G. B., Meijer, C. J., et al. (1992). Prevalence and expression of human papillomavirus in tonsillar carcinomas, indicating a possible viral etiology. *International Journal of Cancer, 51*, 845–850.

Strome, S. E., Savva, A., Brissett, A. E., Gostout, B. S., Lewis, J., Clayton, A. C., et al. (2002). Squamous cell carcinoma of the tonsils: A molecular analysis of HPV associations. *Clinical Cancer Research, 8*, 1093–1100.

Additional References

Anderson, S. R., & Sinacori, J. T. (2007). Plummer-Vinson syndrome heralded by postcricoid carcinoma. *American Journal of Otolaryngology, 28*, 22–24.

Gillison, M. L., & Shah, K. V. (2001). Human papillomavirus-associated head and neck squamous cell carcinoma: Mounting evidence for an etiologic role for human papillomavirus in a subset of head and neck cancers. *Current Opinion in Oncology, 13*, 183–188.

Hammarstedt, L., Lindquist, D., Dahlstrand, H., Romanitan, M., Dahlgren, L. O., Joneberg, J., et al. (2006). Human papillomavirus as a risk factor for the increase in incidence of tonsillar cancer. *International Journal of Cancer, 119*, 2620–2623.

Hobbs, C. G., Sterne, J. A., Bailey, M., Heyderman, R. S., Birchall, M. A., & Thomas, S. J. (2006). Human papillomavirus and head and neck cancer: A systematic review and meta-analysis. *Clinical Otolaryngology, 31*, 259–266.

Vachin, F., Hans, S., Atlan, D., Brasnu, D., Menard, M., & Laccourreye, O. (2004). Long-term results of exclusive chemotherapy for glottic squamous cell carcinoma complete clinical responders after induction chemotherapy. *Annales d'Otolaryngologie et de Chirurgie Cervico-Faciale, 121*, 140–147.

2

MEETING THE CHALLENGES OF TREATMENT PLANNING AND SURGERY FOR HEAD AND NECK CANCER

Eugene N. Myers, MD, FACS FRCS Edin (Hon.)

Part I

Determining Treatment for Oral and Head and Neck Cancer

Squamous cell carcinoma arises from the surface cells of the skin and the mucous membrane lining of the mouth, throat, and voice box (larynx) and is the most common form of head and neck cancer. Skin cancer (squamous cell, basal cell, and malignant melanoma) arises in response to long-term sun exposure. Squamous cell cancer of the mucous membrane usually occurs in individuals with a history of long-term tobacco and alcohol consumption. In recent years evidence suggests that a virus may be the cause of cancer involving the tonsil and tongue base in nonsmoking patients. The identified viruses, human papilloma virus subtypes 16 and 18, are also found in cases of cervical cancers in women (Myers & Suen, 2003).

Other forms of cancer, such as malignant melanoma and adenocarcinoma, may arise from the mucous membranes. Lymphomas can arise from the tonsil, the base of the tongue, the nasopharynx, or lymph nodes in the neck.

Cancer of the head and neck is usually diagnosed at an advanced stage (Ridge, Glisson, Horwitz, & Lango, 2005) for several reasons. One is that the symptoms produced by head and neck cancer are similar to those associated with benign conditions such as sore throat, hoarseness, ear pain, nasal discharge, and swelling in the neck. Another reason for delay in diagnosis is that some patients are in denial about their symptoms and don't go to their doctor or dentist. Patients who do seek treatment may manage their symptoms for extended periods with various medications until the cancer is advanced.

Individuals with cancer arising in the mucous membranes present with a variety of symptoms. Patients with cancer of the vocal cords present with hoarseness. Other symptoms include sore throat, difficulty swallowing, coughing up blood, and aspiration (food going into the windpipe when swallowing) (Ridge et al.,

2005). Patients may experience progressive shortness of breath or complete airway obstruction requiring opening of the neck and placement of a breathing tube (tracheostomy).

Ear pain (otalgia) reflects "referred pain" secondary to cancer invading local nerves that supply innervation to the ear. Unfortunately some patients are mistakenly treated for an ear infection without having a thorough head and neck examination.

Patients with cancer of the tongue or beneath the tongue (floor of the mouth) complain of soreness in these areas, which may progress to difficulty with swallowing (accompanied by weight loss) or with articulation (forming certain words). Some patients will complain of spitting out blood. Some may also have ear pain. Patients may present with difficulty opening the mouth (trismus). Patients with this problem have difficulty with eating and experience marked weight loss.

Cancer of the tonsil and base of the tongue may not have any local symptoms but may present with a lump in one or both sides of the neck. This lump represents spread of the cancer into the lymph nodes of the neck.

Nasopharyngeal cancer is usually seen in Asian people and is rare in Caucasians. Symptoms include hearing loss, nasal obstruction, and a lump in the neck. In advanced cases, destruction of the base of the skull can cause symptoms related to loss of normal nerve function.

When the patient's primary care physician (PCP) or dentist suspects cancer, the patient should be referred to a head and neck surgeon (Ridge et al., 2005). Current treatment is often multimodal, or delivered by more than one doctor, but the surgeon should be responsible for making appropriate referrals to other team members. These other members may include medical oncologists, radiation oncologists, oral maxillofacial surgeons, a maxillofacial prosthodontist, a nutritionist, a social worker, a psychiatrist, specialized nurses, speech and swallowing therapists, hospice, and clergy.

A comprehensive history should be taken, including general health considerations (comorbidities), for example, problems with heart, lungs, liver, diabetes, and HIV. Addictions such as cigarette smoking, alcohol consumption, and narcotics must be revealed because, when present, these may have a profound effect on the immediate or long-term care.

A thorough physical examination must include the skin, mouth, voice box, throat, nasopharynx, and neck. Tumor diagrams should be used to record the location and the size of the tumor. Cancer of the mouth tends to be ulcerated and may have a bad odor. The neck must be thoroughly examined to detect lumps that may contain cancer. The head and neck surgeon will evaluate the extent of invasion below the surface into the deep tissues. The teeth and gums must be examined because patients who smoke and drink heavily may also have cavities and gum (periodontal) disease. A flexible tube with a light on the end may be placed through the nose into the pharynx to examine the pharynx and larynx in detail and to take photos. This procedure is called flexible endoscopy.

To fully evaluate the areas involved by the cancer, imaging studies such as ultrasound, CT scan, or MRI may be necessary. Recently the PET-CT scan has become popular for initial staging purposes and then later to reevaluate the patient, especially those who have received chemoradiation (Fukui, Blodgett, Snyderman, Johnson, & Myers, 2005). These studies are done on an outpatient basis and usually involve an intravenous injection of contrast fluid, which helps the radiologist evaluate the areas of interest. On the basis of physical examination and/or the scan, a fine needle aspiration biopsy (FNAB) may be necessary to obtain a sample of cells for analysis. This may be done in either the doctor's office or another location, with ultrasound guidance. A cancer of the skin, lip, or mouth may be biopsied in the surgeon's office under local anesthesia.

Once the workup is complete, the patient's cancer is "staged" (Gluckman & Wolfe, 2006). The staging system is based on certain criteria, including the size of the primary tumor (T), status of the lymph nodes (N), and any evidence of distant spread, or metastases (M). The TNM system is helpful in guiding treatment options and is a valuable means for members of the health care team to communicate in determining prognosis.

Patients with cancer of the mucous membranes should have an examination and biopsy under general anesthesia. This allows a thorough evaluation without the usual gagging or pain (or both) associated with examination in the doctor's office. A preliminary examination by the patient's family doctor or hospital anesthesiologist will determine the patient's suitability to undergo the examination under anesthesia. An EKG, chest x-ray, and laboratory data are obtained and the patient's condition is optimized prior to anesthesia to prevent complications. The endoscopy will also help to determine the presence of other cancers, which should be incorporated into the treatment program. Patients with bad teeth and gum infection should have dental extractions to allow better healing and to avoid complications after surgery and radiation.

The question of whether cancer of the head and neck should be treated by surgery alone, surgery followed by radiation therapy, or surgery followed by radiation therapy and chemotherapy can be confusing to the patient. Patients must be informed of all treatment options, including no treatment.

When the patient is contemplating surgery, there is a need for a thorough discussion with the surgeon concerning risks and benefits of the procedure. This discussion should also include whether the surgery is outpatient or inpatient and the approximate length of hospital stay. The possible need for surgical reconstruction is an important issue. Reconstruction is usually carried out immediately following the removal of the cancer and thus increases the length of time of the procedure and the hospital stay. Patients with serious medical problems such as chronic lung disease or heart problems may be predisposed to serious, postoperative complications.

Upon the patient's discharge from the hospital, strong family support is ideal but may not be sustainable. In such cases an appropriate long-term care facility becomes a priority. If this phase of rehabilitation is not satisfactory, a growing sense of despair may develop in the patient and lead to a frank depression, making the completion of therapy and reentry into society difficult (Gluckman & Wolfe, 2006). Issues such as pain management and adequate nutritional support must also be addressed.

Part II

Surgical Procedures for Specific Oral and Head and Neck Cancers

The extent of surgery for oral and head and neck cancer depends upon the size and the location of the primary cancer. Early cancers such as those limited to the vocal cord (T_1) are often treated with CO_2 laser. This brief operation is carried out in the hospital on an outpatient basis with the patient under general anesthesia. Little pain is involved, although some muscle soreness in the shoulder and back of the neck may be expected. Patients are usually required to rest their voice and to be on acid reflux medication to ensure good healing.

Patients with more locally advanced cancer of the larynx may be treated with "conservation surgery." These voice-sparing procedures are done through the neck with the voice being conserved in many cases. A tracheostomy (a temporary opening in the windpipe) is required and remains in place for several weeks to allow for swelling of the remaining voice box to subside. Intravenous fluids are given for the first few days, after which nutrition is delivered through a tube, either placed through the nose or inserted directly into the stomach (PEG or gastrostomy tube). Once the patient can breathe sufficiently with the tracheostomy tube plugged, the tube can be removed. Swallowing rehabilitation can then be started with the help of a speech-language pathologist or swallowing coach (dysphagia coach) (Wasserman, Murry, Johnson, & Myers, 2001). Once patients can swallow and maintain their nutritional status, the feeding tube can be removed and the patient discharged.

Patients who progress slowly may be discharged to a skilled nursing facility. The surgeon should then follow the patient, remove the gastrostomy and tracheostomy tubes at the appropriate time, and proceed with swallowing therapy. Pressures to discharge patients as early as possible will result in a modification of this plan, with the discharge likely to take place within the first few days and tube removal and swallowing therapy done on an outpatient basis. Patients undergoing advanced laser surgery usually do not require a tracheotomy or insertion of a feeding tube. The quality of life following these surgical procedures to conserve the voice is usually good.

A total laryngectomy is advised for patients who have advanced local cancer that makes it impossible to save any part of the voice box. A neck dissection is usually included. The same applies to patients who have gone through a full course of radiation therapy or chemotherapy in whom the treatment was not successful. Although a small number of these patients may be eligible for conservation surgery to preserve the voice, patients who are elderly or who have poor lung function or advanced cardiovascular disease are usually advised to have their entire voice box removed. While conservation surgery may be technically feasible, the patient may lack the will or the strength to be successfully rehabilitated and may become dependent on the tracheotomy tube and a stomach tube for feeding. The quality of life under these circumstances is not as good as that with total laryngectomy.

After the total laryngectomy, the throat muscles are sewn together to form a tube so that the patient can swallow normally. Radiation therapy given preoperatively changes the quality of the tissues, which may result in delayed healing. On occasion, the edges of the swallowing passage may partially separate, producing leakage of saliva into the neck with resultant infection draining to the outside, forming a *fistula*. Small fistulas are treated by packing medicated gauze into the opening until the leakage stops. A larger or prolonged leak often requires surgical closure.

After the voice box has been removed, a small opening is made in the back wall of the windpipe into the food passage and a rubber tube is inserted. This tube is removed approximately 2 weeks later and a valve is inserted, which enables the patient to speak when the stoma (hole in the neck) is covered with the thumb. Some surgeons prefer to puncture the windpipe and insert the valve at a later date after all the tissues have healed (Smith & Myers, 2002).

Once the tissue is sufficiently healed, patients may resume their usual activities with a good quality of life. A stoma cover may be used during the day and can be obtained by contacting the Web site of the International Association of Laryngectomees (IAL) at www.larynxlink.com.

The pharynx surrounds the voice box. Cancers that arise in this area may require removal of all or part of the voice box. Removal of the voice box requires surgical reconstruction to permit swallowing. Several choices are available to accomplish this. Skin or muscle from the chest (a flap), which includes its own arteries and veins, is folded to form a tube and sewn to the remaining parts of the throat. In more recent years, an alternative approach has been developed using a "free flap" or "free tissue transfer" in which skin from the forearm or thigh or a portion of the small intestine (jejunum) is removed, together with its own arteries and veins, and transferred as a tube and sewn into the remaining parts of the throat. The arteries and veins of the free flap are sewn to the arteries and veins in the neck. If a free flap from the forearm is used, a skin graft resurfaces the donor site on the arm. In the case of an intestinal flap, the bowel defect is closed without a graft (Fukui et al., 2005). Provision for a voice valve is also included at the time of surgery. Once swelling has subsided, the patient can swallow, which is the most important aspect in measuring the quality of life in a laryngectomy patient.

Oral cancer can affect the tongue (the most common site), the floor of the mouth, the gums, the roof of the mouth (the palate), and the jawbone (the mandible). Radiation therapy without chemotherapy does not usually play a role in the primary treatment of these cancers for cure but may be used postoperatively. A neck dissection is sometimes included at the time of the removal of the cancer, regardless of whether the lymph nodes are enlarged.

Cancer of the tongue almost always arises on the side or undersurface of the tongue. Surgery to remove a small cancer (partial glossectomy) will also include excision of some surrounding normal tissue to ensure complete tumor removal and allow closure of the cut edges of the tongue with a few stitches. A pathologist examines the edges of the tissue to be certain that all of the cancer cells have been removed. This procedure does not require a tracheostomy or a feeding tube. Patients begin to swallow the night of the surgery and are discharged in about 1 or 2 days once the neck dissection is healed sufficiently.

Removal of more extensive tongue cancers may require a skin graft. The graft is usually taken from the thigh and sewn into the edges of the tongue defect. A thin and pliable free flap from the forearm is an alternative. A tracheostomy is performed and a nasogastric feeding tube is used. In 5 to 7 days, tubes are removed and the patient can be discharged. Normal speech and swallowing are to be expected.

When cancer occurs in the back part of the tongue, it may be necessary to divide the jawbone in the midline and open it up to provide enough room to see the entire cancer and to remove it. The jawbone is then repaired using small metal plates and screws.

The entire tongue is rarely removed (total glossectomy) with a mandatory neck dissection. Following surgery, patients are restricted to a thick liquid and pureed diet. A tube is usually inserted into the stomach (PEG or "G" tube) to provide access to nourishment while patients are learning how to swallow. The tracheostomy tube is plugged but kept in place. Once the patient is swallowing without aspiration, the tracheostomy tube can be removed. Only patients who have good lung function, which enables them to cough effectively, will be able to tolerate this surgery. Compromised patients cannot tolerate this procedure and will require a total laryngectomy to avoid developing aspiration pneumonia. Reconstruction with tissue flaps is usually required in these advanced cases.

Cancer of the floor of the mouth usually occurs in the midline, just under the tongue. These cancers are usually removed through the mouth. If the cancer is in the midline, both sides of the neck are dissected. If the cancer is on one side, only that side of the neck is dissected. If the cancer is very close to or adherent to the jawbone, the bone of the gum (and teeth) must be removed. The excised tissues are examined by the pathologist to be certain that all of the cancer has been removed. The raw surfaces are then reconstructed using a skin graft or a free flap taken from the forearm (radial forearm free flap). The graft is sewn into the defect, and a bolus (bolster) dressing is applied. A tracheostomy and nasogastric (NG) feeding tube are inserted and removed within 5 to 7 days. Patients are able to speak and swallow normally when the healing is complete.

The jawbone (mandible) may be invaded by cancer directly from the soft tissues of the gum or secondarily by cancer of the floor of the mouth/tongue. In advanced cases the skin of the lip, chin, or cheek may also be involved. The approach is usually through an incision in the skin rather than just through the mouth. Neck dissections are always included with this surgery. It is important to remove adequate amounts of what looks like normal bone adjacent to the cancer since the pathologist cannot examine the bone margin under the microscope by frozen section. After removal of the jawbone and necessary skin or tissue of the mouth, reconstruction is carried out. This is particularly true in patients in whom the bone of the chin is involved because failure to reconstruct this area leads to inability to close the mouth or to speak or swallow. The introduction of free tissue flaps containing bone from either the arm or leg allows for jawbone reconstruction. Metal plates and screws are used to fix the bone graft to the remaining jawbone. Tracheostomy and an NG tube are used and are removed once the swelling diminishes and the tissues are healed.

Small cancers of the inside of the cheek may be removed through the mouth. A neck dissection is included. A skin graft is used to resurface the raw area. A bolus dressing holds the skin graft in place. No tracheostomy or NG tube is used in such cases. Patients with more advanced cancers in the cheek may require removal of the overlying skin, when involved, or the jawbone. This requires reconstruction as described previously, with resumption of normal speaking and swallowing expected along with a good quality of life.

Cancer of the roof of the mouth (hard palate) and upper gum is usually squamous cell carcinoma. Cancers (adenocarcinomas) may also arise from minor salivary glands or mucous glands located in the hard palate. The cancer may invade the underlying bone, which must be removed. The separation between the mouth and nose is lost, resulting in food coming out of the nose when the patient swallows and less intelligible speech.

Prior to this type of surgery, the patient must be referred to a maxillofacial prosthodontist (a dentist with special training in making dental appliances, or prostheses) to design and construct a prosthesis to replace the roof of the mouth, restore oral-nasal separation, and allow normal speech and swallowing. Patients with remaining upper teeth will have a prosthesis (obturator), which clips onto the teeth. Patients without teeth have a more difficult time with retention of the prosthesis. Patients with more extensive cancer that requires removal of the surrounding soft tissue, such as the soft palate and tonsil, will benefit from the prosthesis, but speech and swallowing will probably be compromised.

After healing has progressed, a "temporary prosthesis" (without teeth) is made while the tissues become sufficiently healed to accommodate a permanent prosthesis with teeth. Daily oral cleansing with salt water or hydrogen peroxide mixed half and half with water is performed. A water pick is also useful to keep the cavity free of dried mucus. Normal quality of life is expected.

In recent years techniques for palatal reconstruction using free flaps with bone have been devised to eliminate the need for prostheses and to close the surgical defect (Myers & Suen, 2003). On the positive side, a prosthesis is not necessary; on the negative side, the cavity is no longer open for the surgeon to examine and monitor for possible regrowth of the cancer.

Cancer of the head and neck has the potential to spread (metastasize) to the lymph nodes in the neck and may require a radical neck dissection. This procedure consists of removal of all of the lymph nodes in the neck, the jugular vein, as well as the big muscle (sternocleidomastoid) in the neck and spinal accessory nerve that supplies innervation to the shoulder muscle (trapezius). While control of active cancer of the lymph nodes is excellent with this operation, especially when combined with postoperative radiation therapy, there are drawbacks to this procedure, including aesthetics, reduced shoulder function, and decreased range of arm motion.

In more recent years, the concept of the "selective neck dissection," rather than a radical dissection, has become popular (Myers & Gastman, 2003). This operation can be performed in patients without definite positive lymph nodes. If cancer is found, additional treatment with radiation therapy or combined chemoradiation may be given. If all lymph nodes are free of cancer, the patient's chance for cure is better. Patients who have advanced cancer in the neck (very large or partially fixed lymph nodes) will require radical or modified neck dissection.

Patients who have had a selective neck dissection usually have minimal side effects. Alternatively, patients who have had a radical neck dissection must enter into a special physical therapy program, specifically designed to prevent shoulder dysfunction. A diligent exercise program will allow the patient to avoid shoulder pain, marked disability, and a severe cosmetic defect.

Cancers involving the parotid gland are relatively rare. The parotid gland, which produces saliva, is located just in front of or below the ear and usually is associated with benign tumors (80% to 90%). The characteristic sign of a tumor in the parotid gland is a lump. It is difficult to tell benign from malignant; however, if the mass has grown rapidly, is associated with pain or paralysis of the face, it is usually malignant. Cancer of the parotid gland may be low grade and is treated by surgical removal through an incision in front of and below the ear. The facial nerve can usually be preserved with no neck dissection necessary. Although there should be no side effects from the surgery and quality of life should be undisturbed, there may be some cases in which numbness of the lower half of the ear may occur.

Patients with high-grade cancer of the parotid gland, especially if facial paralysis is present, will need a total parotidectomy, removal of the facial nerve, and a neck dissection followed by radiation therapy (Myers & Suen, 2003). Reconstruction of the facial nerve is necessary.

Patients with cancer of the head and neck are under great emotional strain during this time because these operations, while designed to cure cancer, also threaten patients' appearance, function, and life. The first few days after the surgery, the patients are usually quite happy and, in fact, elated and relieved. However, 3 to 4 days postoperatively it is not unusual for the patient to become depressed. This may be due to the realization that they have cancer and that its treatment will impact their lifestyle, and their emotions may be magnified by the loss of interpersonal support systems and the obvious loss, whether temporary or permanent, of the ability to communicate (Lydiatt, 2006). Recognition of this problem by the surgeon; a frank discussion of the fact that this is a natural postoperative event; and a positive attitude on the part of the surgeons, the nursing staff, and the personal caregiver often alleviate these temporary depressive symptoms without the need for medications or psychiatric consultation.

The diagnosis of cancer instantly changes the life of the individual. However, a word should also be said about the caregivers. The patient's loved ones and caregivers may experience emotions similar to those of the patient. They may worry about financial security and how the patient's disability may affect future plans, and they may even become preoccupied with thoughts of death. While a patient experiences the pain of surgery and other forms of cancer treatment, caregivers have a shared pain for the impact of the treatment on the patient and also on their family's structure, lifestyle, and future. There is a need for the entire support system to come into play to cope with these problems (Gluckman & Wolfe, 2006).

Current management involves treatment by a team of professionals. The surgeon, who is usually the first to meet the patient, should be the one to monitor the patient's overall progress. Follow-up visits should be frequent enough to answer the patient's questions about symptoms, including pain, lack of normal function, dry mouth, or need for further treatment or rehabilitation. Close follow-up is also necessary because of the potential for patients with squamous cell carcinoma to develop second primary cancers (15% to 20%). Second primary cancers may occur in the head and neck, lung, or esophagus.

Surgeons and their staffs must be aware not only of the physical needs such as nutrition and pain relief but also of the emotional needs of the patient and the caregiver and the impact on the family unit. They should be willing, able, and available to meet their needs and provide support.

References

Fukui, M. D., Blodgett, T. M., Snyderman, C. H., Johnson, J. T., & Myers, E. N. (2005). Combined PET-CT in the head and neck: Part II, diagnostic uses and pitfalls of oncologic imaging. *Radio Graphics, 25*, 913–930.

Gluckman, J. L., & Wolfe, M. (2006). Head and neck cancer in the geriatric patient. In K. H. Calhoun & D. E. Eibling (Eds.), *Geriatric otolaryngology*. New York: Taylor & Francis.

Lydiatt, W. M. (2006, September). A review of depression in head and neck cancer. *News from SPOHNC.*

Myers, E. N., & Gastman, B. L. (2003). Neck dissection: An operation in evolution. *Archives of Otolaryngology—Head and Neck Surgery, 192,* 14–25.

Myers, E. N., & Suen, J. (2003). *Cancer of the head and neck* (4th ed.). Philadelphia: W. B. Saunders.

Ridge, J. A., Glisson, B. S., Horwitz, E. M., & Lango, M. N. (2005). Head and neck tumors. In R. Pazdur, W. Hoskins, L. Coia, & L. Wagman (Eds.), *Cancer management: A multidisciplinary approach*. Manhasset, NY: Oncology Publishing Group.

Smith, J., & Myers, E. N. (2002). Progress in laryngeal surgery. *Head & Neck, 20,* 955–964.

Wasserman, T., Murry, T., Johnson, J. T., & Myers, E. N. (2001). Management of swallowing in supraglottic and extended supraglottic patients. *Head & Neck, 23,* 1043–1048.

3

MEETING THE CHALLENGES OF RADIATION THERAPY

David M. Brizel, MD,
Mary Ann Downey Rubio, PA-C
Gail Funk, RN, OCN, Linda Gilliard, MS, RD

Nearly 40,000 cases of head and neck cancer are diagnosed annually in the United States. Approximately 90% of these are squamous cell carcinoma. Radiotherapy plays a major role in the treatment of these cancers, either as curative intent therapy or given post-operatively after surgery.

Ionizing radiation enters tissues and forms free radicals within the cell that damage DNA, resulting in cell death. Radiation is a useful treatment because cancer cells are more sensitive to its effects than are normal tissues. Radiation is a localized form of treatment. The most common types of external beam radiation are photons or x-rays, which are capable of deep penetration through tissues, and electrons, where the depth of penetration can be chosen to be superficial or deeper.

Curative intent radiation therapy for stage I and II disease is generally delivered once a day over the course of 7 weeks. Systemic chemotherapy is not typically given for early stage disease. In stage III and IV disease, radiation may be delivered once or twice daily with "concomitant boost" treatment in which the patient starts with once-daily treatment and finishes with twice-daily treatment during the last 2 weeks. Radiation therapy given twice daily for the entire course of treatment may also be used for very large or aggressive tumors. Chemotherapy or targeted therapy given concurrently with radiation is the standard of care for locally advanced stage III/IV disease because it significantly reduces the risk of recurrence and improves the odds of survival. A drug typically used for chemotherapy is cisplatin (Bernier et al., 2004; Bourhis et al., 2006; Brizel et al., 1998; Cooper et al., 2004; Forastiere et al., 2003); for targeted therapy, cetuximab (Erbitux,) is typically used (Bonner et al., 2006). Other drugs may be used routinely or in the setting of clinical trials depending upon which institution is coordinating the treatment. Patient age, performance status, and coexisting medical conditions will drive the physician's treatment recommendations.

Various techniques can be used to deliver external beam radiation for treatment of head and neck cancer. Conventional 2-D, conformal 3-D therapy, intensity modulated radiation therapy (IMRT), and, occasionally, brachytherapy are the most common techniques. Some institutions are investigating the use of protons.

2-D treatment consists of two beams (fields) that evenly deliver radiation from the right and left side of the patient. Commonly, a third beam will be aimed from in front of the patient to irradiate lymph nodes in the lower part of the neck that are not included in the upper fields. Such treatment can very effectively treat tumors but often delivers large doses of radiation to uninvolved structures such as the parotid salivary glands. Consequently, permanent xerostomia (dry mouth) arises in a significant proportion of patients who undergo 2-D treatment. Amifostine (Ethyol,), a drug that can be administered intravenously or subcutaneously prior to each daily dose of radiation, can reduce the incidence and severity of this complication (Brizel et al., 2000). The FDA has approved amifostine for use in the setting of once-daily post-operative irradiation. However, it can cause nausea/vomiting, low blood pressure, and rash. Its benefit in settings where twice-daily radiation or concurrent chemotherapy is used or for the prevention of other complications has not been established.

IMRT and 3-D provide radiation dose distributions that conform much more closely to the shape of the tumor volume. These techniques can more effectively reduce the amount of radiation that is delivered to non-cancerous normal tissues and thus reduce treatment-induced side effects, including xerostomia. They both will commonly use as many as 5 to 11 different beams to achieve this goal, although more beams are typically used with IMRT than 3-D. The size and shape of each individual field will stay constant while the beam is on with 3-D. With IMRT, the field size and shape will change continuously while the beam is on. IMRT is now the standard of care for virtually all academic radiation departments and in most centers with large numbers of head and neck cancer patients.

Brachytherapy (implants) consists of the physical placement of radioisotopes into a tumor to locally deliver radiation. An implant will also deliver a conformal dose distribution. Implants are usually performed in the operating room and only for specialized circumstances. Increasing adoption of IMRT has further reduced the need to perform implants.

Increased sophistication in treatment planning and delivery requires precise, consistent patient immobilization. Typically a head holder is used to achieve this aim. It is a plastic mesh that becomes soft and flexible when soaked in warm water. It is then placed over the face and head and allowed to cool. The mesh hardens and retains shape during treatment. The head holder is clamped to the table when it is first made during treatment simulation and again during each radiation treatment. Breathing through the mask is not difficult, but claustrophobic or anxious patients may require a short-acting anti-anxiety medication.

Treatment and management of the patient with head and neck cancer requires an integrated multidisciplinary team consisting of the radiation oncologist, medical oncologist, head and neck surgeon, dentist, mid-level practitioner (physician assistants and nurse practitioners), nurse, nutritionist, social worker, speech pathologist, counselor, dosimetrist, physicist, and other therapists.

The side effects of treatment are classified as either acute or late. The former are those that occur during treatment and that may persist for 2–3 months after the completion of radiotherapy. The latter are those that typically arise after recovery from the acute side effects. Patients are at risk for the development of late side effects for the remainder of their lives. The type and severity of side effects depend upon the type and location of the tumor, the radiation technique used and the dose delivered, and whether or not chemotherapy is administered. The physician and team are well aware of these side effects, their usual time and mode of presentation, and the appropriate management to preserve patient functional status to the greatest extent possible.

Adequate nutrition before, during, and after radiotherapy is crucial to the successful completion of treatment and to proper healing after radiation is completed. Head and neck radiotherapy causes side effects that will impair nutritional intake. Early professional dietary intervention with a registered dietitian will help to improve quality of life and recovery from treatment side effects (Larsson, Hedelin, Johansson, & Athlin, 2005; Dawson, Morley, Robertson, & Soutar, 2001; Munshi et al., 2003; Colasanto, Prasad, Nash, Decker, & Wilson, 2005; Dixon, 2004). By increasing the probability of successfully completing treatment, overall chances for survival will increase. If weight loss has occurred at the time of diagnosis, it is very important that dietary interventions be implemented to discourage further weight loss. The initial step is to determine the cause of weight loss. If lower intake is due to a loss of appetite, then education on making foods calorically dense in small quantities and eating more frequently throughout the day will encourage weight maintenance. If chewing and swallowing certain textures has become difficult, then eating softer foods and liquids that are dense with calories is the goal. Nutritional drinks such as Ensure Plus, Boost Plus, or Carnation Instant Breakfast are beneficial supplements to the diet. If there has been no weight loss prior to radiotherapy, then continuing to maintain weight throughout treatment is the goal.

Monitoring weight closely by using the same scale at the same time of day, several days per week will help to discourage rapid weight loss. Adding an appropriate snack or supplement or making foods calorically dense are necessary dietary changes that should be made if weight loss occurs at any point during treatment. If weight maintenance is not possible by eating and drinking, a feeding tube should be placed. In patients who are having nutritional problems or are anticipating major nutritional problems, the feeding tube should be placed prior to beginning radiation therapy, especially if chemotherapy is to be part of the treatment. Intensive, professional nutritional support and aggressive management of pain by physicians and nurses during treatment will help patients avoid a feeding tube.

Following is a discussion of side effects that patients can experience during therapy. The type and location of the tumor, the radiation technique used, and the administration of concurrent chemotherapy will determine the type and severity of these side effects.

Skin reactions may occur 3 to 4 weeks into therapy and range from skin redness (grade 1) to moist desquamation or shedding of the outer layers of the skin (grade 3). Keeping the area clean with gentle soap and water, protected with lotions that do not contain alcohol, and avoiding tight clothing that will rub and further irritate the area are key. Patients should not apply lotions in the 4 hours prior to treatment; however, they may be applied as needed after treatment. Skin reaction generally resolves within 10 days after completion of radiotherapy.

Mouth pain, throat pain, or painful swallowing is variable in onset and highly dependent on type and location of tumor as well as radiation technique. Generally, symptoms become noticeable within 2 weeks of the initiation of radiotherapy. These symptoms are collectively referred to as mucositis. They are severe in at least 50% of patients who receive radiation with concurrent chemotherapy. Local anesthetics such as over-the-counter Sucrets, Chloroseptic, or prescription viscous lidocaine are used initially, followed by anti-inflammatories and then narcotic pain medication. The goal of management is to keep pain below a 3 on the 0–10 pain scale (10 being "unbearable"). Generally, a patient with a pain level greater than 3 will be unable to eat and drink in a manner that allows maintenance of weight and/or hydration. Consequently, IV fluid rehydration may become necessary, or feeding tube placement into the stomach may be required.

Thickened saliva/dry mouth is one of the major long-term quality-of-life issues associated with head and neck radiation therapy. This can be temporary or permanent and varies in severity depending on the location of the tumor and radiation technique. IMRT has significantly reduced the incidence of long-term xerostomia after treatment. Altered saliva predisposes patients to oral fungal infection and tooth decay. It is of utmost importance that all patients with head and neck cancer who will undergo radiation therapy have a thorough dental evaluation prior to the start of treatments with frequent follow-up care and emphasis on preventive dental care.

During therapy the saliva typically gets thick and ropey, finally progressing to dry mouth. There are a number of over-the-counter artificial saliva products available that will help with dry mouth. When the saliva is thick and ropey, a solution of 1:3 parts peroxide and water used as a gargle will help break up the mucus so it is easily cleared. Additionally, guaifenesin, an over-the-counter mucolytic or thinning agent, serves to thin secretions so they may be cleared. This comes in liquid and pill form but must be taken with increased fluid to be effective.

Following completion of radiation, routine dental evaluation and cleaning should be performed every 3 to 4 months to reduce the risk of secondary sequelae of xerostomia. If dry mouth is severe and not responsive to artificial saliva products, there are a few medications that can be prescribed, including pilocarpine (Salagen®) and cevimeline (Evoxac®). They are beneficial to 30% to 50% of patients, but they have side effects and cannot be taken if the patient has certain heart problems, emphysema, or glaucoma.

Other side effects of treatment may include:

- Loss of taste and appetite generally occurs as the changes in saliva occur and may persist for up to 6 weeks following completion of therapy. The return of taste may not be what it was prior to diagnosis and treatment.
- Fatigue will range from mild to profound. A patient will be examined each week during therapy and queried for this because some contributing conditions, such as low blood count, are easily evaluated and treated.
- The occurrence of nausea or dizziness is dependent on radiation technique and tumor location. These symptoms are also easily treated and resolve with completion of treatment.
- Loss of hair, either temporary or permanent, may occur within the treatment field.

Some late effects that have been observed include dry mouth, possible dental decay, osteoradionecrosis (death of bone tissue) or radiation-induced soft tissue necrosis, carotid artery stenosis (narrowing), scarring or edema of structures in the treatment field, and, though rarely, the risk of radiation-induced second malignancy. Any of these side effects should be discussed with a physician.

Radiation therapy is the standard nonsurgical treatment for oral head and neck cancer. Concurrent chemotherapy and radiation therapy is the standard of treatment when surgical options carry significant functional morbidity or when the tumor is unresectable. Treatment demands a multidisciplinary team, expert in the delivery of therapy. Improvements in technology have increased the chances of cure, but compliance with treatment is paramount to the likelihood of success. The multidisciplinary team also plays a crucial role in facilitating compliance via the skilled management of the various side effects that occur with treatment.

References

Bernier, J., Domenge, C., Ozsahin M., Matuszewska, K., Lefebvre, J. L., Greiner, R. H., et al. (2004). Postoperative irradiation with or without concomitant chemotherapy for locally advanced head and neck cancer. *New England Journal of Medicine, 350,* 1945–1952.

Bonner, J. A., Harari, P. M., Giralt, J., Azarnia, N., Shin, D., Cohen, R., et al. (2006). Radiotherapy plus cetuximab for squamous-cell carcinoma of the head and neck. *New England Journal of Medicine, 354,* 567–578.

Bourhis, J., Overgaard, J., Audry, H., Ang, K. K., Saunders, M., Bernier, J., et al. (2006). Hyperfractionated or accelerated radiotherapy in head and neck cancer: A meta-analysis. *Lancet, 368,* 843–854.

Brizel, D. M., Albers, M. E., Fisher, S. R., Scher, R. L., Richtsmeier, W. J., Hars, V., et al. (1998). Hyperfractionated irradiation with or without concurrent chemotherapy for locally advanced head and neck cancer. *New England Journal of Medicine, 338,* 1798–1804.

Brizel, D. M., Wasserman, T. H., Henke, M., Strnad, V., Rudat, V., Monnier, A., et al. (2000). Phase III randomized trial of amifostine as a radioprotector in head and neck cancer. *Journal of Clinical Oncology, 18,* 3339–3345.

Colasanto, J. M., Prasad, P., Nash, M. A., Decker, R. H., & Wilson, L. D. (2005). Nutritional support of patients undergoing radiation therapy for head and neck cancer. *Oncology, 19*(3), 371–379.

Cooper, J. S., Pajak, T. F., Forastiere, A. A., Jacobs, J., Campbell, B. H., Saxman, S. B., et al. (2004). Postoperative concurrent radiotherapy and chemotherapy for high-risk squamous-cell carcinoma of the head and neck. *New England Journal of Medicine, 350,* 1937–1944.

Dawson, E. R., Morley, S. E., Robertson, A. G., & Soutar, D. S. (2001). Increasing dietary supervision can reduce weight loss in oral cancer patients. *Nutrition and Cancer, 41*(1&2), 70–74.

Dixon, S. (2004). Head and neck management: Importance of nutrition intervention. *Oncology Nutrition Connection, 12*(3), 1–11.

Forastiere, A. A., Goepfert, H., Maor, M., Pajak, T. F., Weber, R., Morrison, W., et al. (2003). Concurrent chemotherapy and radiotherapy for organ preservation in advanced laryngeal cancer. *New England Journal of Medicine, 349,* 2091–2098.

Larsson, M., Hedelin, B., Johansson, I., & Athlin, E. (2005). Eating problems and weight loss for patients with head and neck cancer: A chart review from diagnosis until one year after diagnosis. *Cancer Nursing, 28*(6), 425–435.

Munshi, A., Pandey, M. B., Durga, T., Pandey, K. C., Bahadur, S., & Mohanti, B. K. (2003). Weight loss during radiotherapy for head and neck malignancies: What factors impact it? *Nutrition and Cancer, 47*(2), 136–140.

4

MEETING THE CHALLENGES OF CHEMOTHERAPY IN THE TREATMENT OF ORAL AND HEAD AND NECK CANCER

Su Hsien Lim, MD
Matthew Fury, MD, PhD
David G. Pfister, MD

Treating Head and Neck Squamous Cell Carcinoma with Chemotherapy

Historically, surgery and radiation have been the cornerstones of treatment for head and neck squamous cell cancers (HNSCC), especially when the disease is limited to above the collarbones and cure is possible. Chemotherapy alone rarely leads to a cure for these tumors and has been used in the past mainly for patients in whom disease has recurred or spread to a distant site, in hopes of prolonging survival and relieving symptoms. However, the results of clinical trials over the past 20 years have provided the basis for a much greater role for chemotherapy and clarified both when and how to use drug therapy with radiation and surgery to improve disease control.

What Is Chemotherapy and Why Is It Given?

Cancer develops when cells in a part of the body begin to grow in an abnormal and uncontrolled manner. Chemotherapy is drug treatment that is used to try to either control the multiplication or kill these abnormal cancer cells, thus causing tumors to shrink and preventing their spread. When it is given along with other treatments, such as radiation, chemotherapy can also improve the effectiveness of those treatments.

There are many different types of chemotherapy drugs that work by interfering with various parts of a cancer cell's internal structure and function or the process of cell division or duplication. Newer "targeted" agents, including monoclonal antibodies (proteins designed to target a specific site on the cancer cell) and hormonal treatments work by affecting very specific metabolic processes.

How and When Is Chemotherapy Used in the Treatment of Head and Neck Cancer?

There are several different indications for the use of chemotherapy in the treatment of HNSCC.

Treatment of Locally or Regionally Advanced Disease

Locoregionally advanced disease is defined as large primary tumors or tumors with spread to neck lymph nodes that have not spread beyond the head and neck region. These cancers are treated with the intention of cure, but the prognosis is worse than in patients with less advanced disease. Historically, the treatment approach for these advanced cancers has depended on whether surgery was possible. When operable, patients generally underwent surgery followed by postoperative radiation therapy. However, surgery in this setting may lead to altered facial appearance and difficulties with key functions such as speaking, chewing, and swallowing despite advances in surgical techniques and reconstruction. Larger tumors that could not be surgically removed were treated with radiation alone with disappointing cure rates.

In these patients with locoregionally advanced disease, chemotherapy can be used with surgery and/or radiation in three main ways: concurrently (at the same time) with radiation, as adjuvant therapy (after surgery or radiation), or as induction/neoadjuvant therapy (before other treatment).

- ◼ *Concurrent chemoradiation*, or chemotherapy given at the same time as radiation therapy, has proved to be more effective than radiation alone at disease control for tumors that cannot be surgically removed (Brizel et al., 1998; Adelstein et al., 2003; Fountzilas et al., 2004), including advanced nasopharyngeal carcinoma (Al-Sarraf et al., 1998), advanced oropharyngeal cancer (Calais et al., 1999), and in the adjuvant setting after surgery in patients with disease at high risk for relapse as discussed next (Bernier et al., 2004; Cooper et al., 2004). It also achieves a better rate of organ preservation, such as preservation of the voice box, than radiotherapy alone (Forastiere et al., 2006), offering patients the option of avoiding surgery without compromise in cure rates.

- ◼ *Adjuvant therapy*, or therapy given after primary treatment, is used when patients are found at surgery to have high-risk pathological features (that is, features in their tumors worrisome for more aggressive disease and associated with a greater likelihood of recurrence). The addition of adjuvant therapy decreases the risk of relapse. Historically, adjuvant treatment has been with radiation therapy alone; chemotherapy alone has not been shown to improve survival. However, recent studies have found that the addition of cisplatin chemotherapy concurrently with radiation therapy significantly improves disease control above the collarbones in patients at a higher risk of relapse (Bernier et al., 2004; Cooper et al., 2004). On a collective analysis of both studies, two pathological features were particularly associated with benefit from the incorporation of chemotherapy: the presence of cancer cells at the surgical margins (positive margins), or the extension of tumor cells outside of lymph nodes into the surrounding tissue (extracapsular spread or extension) (Bernier et al., 2005).

■ *Neoadjuvant therapy*, or chemotherapy given prior to definitive therapy with either surgery and/or radiation to the primary site and neck, was the focus of several randomized clinical trials during the 1980s and 1990s. Although tumors can demonstrate significant shrinkage, and the incidence of distant metastases may decrease with the use of induction chemotherapy, a collective analysis of these studies (meta-analysis) failed to demonstrate a convincing benefit to overall survival with the addition of chemotherapy in this manner (Pignon, Bourhis, Domenge, & Designe, 2000).

However, there is renewed interest in induction/neoadjuvant therapy for two reasons. First, more effective treatment for locoregional disease has resulted in better control of tumors above the collarbones, such that the development of metastatic disease to other sites in the body has become a more common type of treatment failure. Induction chemotherapy is one way to potentially decrease the rate of these distant metastases. Second, newer triplet combination chemotherapy regimens (either docetaxel or paclitaxel, combined with cisplatin and 5-fluororuacil) appear more effective than the historically used doublet of cisplatin and 5-fluorouracil alone (Hitt et al., 2005; Posner et al, 2007, Vermorken, Remenar et al., 2007). Studies comparing concurrent chemoradiation alone to induction triplet chemotherapy followed by chemoradiation are in progress to determine whether the latter approach improves survival compared with the former one and to what extent the toxicity of treatment is also increased.

Treatment of Recurrent or Metastatic Disease

Locoregionally recurrent HNSCC refers to disease that has come back in the head and neck area but has not spread anywhere else in the body. In this case, surgery and/or radiation may be used with the intent of cure and is successful to this end in selected patients. If neither surgery nor radiation is possible for new locoregional relapse, or if the cancer is metastatic by having spread to other body regions, then the prognosis is much worse. Selected patients may benefit from surgical removal of a distant site of disease, particularly if limited to the lungs, but chemotherapy alone is more commonly used in this situation. The goals of treatment are prolongation of life, decrease in symptoms, and improvement in quality of life. These patients, on average, live less than a year.

First-line therapy in the recurrent or metastatic setting often consists of a platinum-based doublet. Commonly used examples include cisplatin combined with other drugs active in HNSCC such as paclitaxel or 5-fluorouracil. The rates of major tumor shrinkage seen with these treatments are approximately 30% to 40%, but the duration is generally measured in weeks to months, and a significant survival advantage compared with treatment with single drugs that have lower response rates but also lower side effects is not well established (Cohen, Lingen, & Vokes, 2004). Second-line therapies typically employ a single agent, offer lower response rates, and have a disappointing impact with regard to prolonging survival (Leon et al., 2005).

What Types of Chemotherapy Are Being Used Today?

Active classic chemotherapeutic agents for HNSCC include, but are not limited to, methotrexate, cisplatin, carboplatin, 5-fluorouracil, paclitaxel, docetaxel, gemcitabine, and bleomycin. Each of these drugs works differently to control the growth, multiplication, and survival of cancer cells. The anticipated rates of major tumor shrinkage in the relapsed or metastatic disease setting when a single drug is used are approximately 10% to 20%; using a combination of drugs doubles the major response rates. The tumor shrinkage rates further improve when drugs are used as the initial (induction/neoadjuvant) treatment prior to surgery or radiation.

Given the somewhat disappointing effectiveness of the current chemotherapy for recurrent or metastatic HNSCC, there is much ongoing research to identify new and better drugs. There is particular interest in agents that look to exploit newly identified molecular targets in cancer cells and thus offer the hope for treatment that is more specific to the tumor and less toxic to the noncancerous normal tissue and the patient targeted therapies. Cetuximab is an example of such a drug. Cetuximab is a monoclonal antibody that targets the epidermal growth factor receptor (EGFR), a structure expressed on most HNSCC cells involved in the growth and spread of disease. Cetuximab was approved by the Food and Drug Administration in 2006 for use in the primary treatment of HNSCC concurrently with radiation as well as for recurrent or metastatic disease that no longer responds to cisplatin. Preliminary data from a recent study indicate that it provides added anticancer effect when combined with a platinum-based doublet in the first-line setting (Vermorken, Mesia et al., 2007).

Another example of an area of interest for targeted cancer treatment is the development of drugs that interfere with the process of angiogenesis (the creation of blood vessels that feed the tumor). Angiogenesis is promoted by vascular endothelial growth factor (VEGF). Bevacizumab is an example of an antiangiogenesis therapy, being an antibody that binds to VEGF and prevents it from inducing blood vessel growth into tumors. Unlike cetuximab, bevacizumab is not currently approved by the Food and Drug Administration for the treatment of HNSCC.

How Are Chemotherapy Drugs Given?

Most commonly, chemotherapy is delivered directly into the bloodstream through an intravenous catheter. The drug is typically diluted in intravenous fluid prior to administration. Increasingly, chemotherapy is becoming available in oral form as a pill or capsule.

Although a single chemotherapy drug can be given, different drugs are frequently given in combination. The rationale for this strategy is to reduce the chance that the cancer cells will be resistant or will develop resistance to the drugs administered. However, when multiple drugs are given, the side effects are usually greater.

Chemotherapy is frequently administered in cycles. The length of the cycle varies depending on the drug and the regimen. These cycle lengths have been previously determined based on the way the body metabolizes the drugs and prior studies. Depending on the agent or drug combination, dosing may range from daily administration to treatment every 3 to 4 weeks, with time off given in between cycles.

The overall duration of a course of chemotherapy will vary. Sometimes it is set, for example, with induction/neoadjuvant, concurrent, or adjuvant therapy, when a specified number of therapy cycles are planned. Other times, such as when the principal intent of treatment is not to cure but rather to decrease symptoms, it is given until maximum response occurs or limiting side effects develop, which typically happens within 4 to 6 months. Response to chemotherapy is generally assessed by physical exam or imaging approximately every 2 months. If tumor growth occurs, a change in therapy is indicated.

What Are the Side Effects of Chemotherapy and What Can Be Done to Minimize and Alleviate Them?

Chemotherapy targets rapidly growing or dividing cells. This includes not only the cancers cells but also normal cells such as hair follicles, the cells lining the gastrointestinal tract, reproductive cells (sperm), and blood-forming cells. Side effects from chemotherapy are caused by the disruption of the proper function of these cells. Patients may experience alopecia (hair loss), diarrhea, nausea, mouth sores, decreased fertility, increased risk of infection, anemia, bleeding, and generalized fatigue and weakness.

Specific drugs have their own side effects in addition to the more general side effects of chemotherapy. Examples may include nerve effects manifested as numbness and tingling of the hands and feet, hearing loss and ringing in the ears, decline in the kidney's function, decline in the heart's function, damage to the liver, rash, and derangements in the blood's ability to clot.

In addition, there is the risk of a hypersensitivity or allergic reaction to some chemotherapies. Symptoms of hypersensitivity range from mild effects such as rash to rare but life-threatening ones such as shock. For chemotherapy drugs that are prone to cause hypersensitivity, pretreatment with certain medications such as antihistamines and steroids is employed. If a reaction nonetheless occurs, additional medication will be administered or use of that particular chemotherapy may need to be discontinued.

The extent of side effects experienced by any one patient varies. Several different drugs and approaches can be used to minimize and alleviate the side effects. Nausea and vomiting can be minimized with the use of drugs before or after treatment. Examples include dexamethasone (a steroid); aprepitant; and 5-HT_3 receptor antagonists such as palonosetron, ondansetron, dolasetron, granisetron, and alosetron. Other antinausea medicines are given as needed, such as metoclopramide, prochlorperazine, and lorazepam.

The blood count is monitored very closely in patients undergoing chemotherapy, and if the number of cells is too low, chemotherapy may be held or postponed. Colony-stimulating agents are proteins that the body produces to induce production of certain blood components that can now be manufactured for external administration. Erythropoetin or darbepoetin may be administered if the red blood cell count is low and the patient is experiencing fatigue, weakness, or shortness of breath but is not recommended concurrently during radiation treatment because the effectiveness of therapy may be adversely affected (Henke et al., 2003). Granulocyte colony-stimulating factor (e.g., filgrastim) may be administered for a low white blood cell count or as a preventive measure if the course of chemotherapy to be given is known to significantly suppress the white blood cell count.

Other drugs are given to minimize the side effects of radiation treatment. Amifostine is sometimes given during treatment to decrease the incidence of acute and chronic dry mouth (Brizel et al., 2000) but can be associated with side effects of its own (e.g., nausea and low blood pressure). Pilocarpine and cevimeline have been found to improve saliva production and symptoms of dry mouth as well (Johnson et al., 1993; Chambers et al., 2007).

To minimize toxicity to the kidneys from certain chemotherapy drugs, adequate fluid intake is ensured by infusion of saline prior to, during, and after administration of chemotherapy. Furthermore, it is confirmed prior to the start of treatment that the patient has a good urine output to make sure the drug will be cleared by the kidneys. Kidney function is also monitored, and if the kidney demonstrates disturbances in its ability to regulate and retain the electrolytes (minerals such as potassium and magnesium) that the body requires, supplementation of particular electrolytes may be necessary. If there is persistent deterioration in kidney function, the offending chemotherapeutic drug may need to be decreased or stopped.

Damage to the nerves resulting in neuropathy is associated with certain chemotherapies. Vitamin supplementation may help (e.g., vitamin B_{12}). Also, certain medications may decrease the severity of symptoms (e.g., amitriptyline and pregabalin). However, if the neuropathy becomes debilitating, the chemotherapy drug is usually stopped.

Dose-dependent cardiac toxicity is uncommon except with doxorubicin, a drug that is used in the treatment of certain types of thyroid cancers but not typically HNSCC. During treatment heart function is closely monitored through echocardiograms. To maximize the amount of chemotherapy that can be delivered, a special formulation of doxorubicin (liposomal doxorubicin) or a cardioprotective agent such as dexrazoxane can be used (Shah, Lincoff, & Young, 1996).

Certain drugs may cause inflammation of the liver. Patients with significant liver involvement by the cancer may be more vulnerable to this side effect because they often have a less normally functioning liver when they start treatment, although this is uncommon in head and neck cancers. Regular blood tests are performed to check on the function of the liver. Intake of substances potentially toxic to the liver, such as acetaminophen and alcohol, should be minimized and monitored during treatment.

Chemotherapy may result in temporary or permanent sterility (inability to have children). In men, this is caused by a decline or cessation in sperm production; in women, this is due to changes in the menstrual cycle resulting in irregular or infrequent menses. Menopause may occur in some women who are perimenopausal. In younger women the menstrual cycle often resumes and fertility returns. Many men choose to bank their sperm in anticipation of receiving chemotherapy. Because of concerns regarding the teratogenic effects (causing malformations and defects to the fetus) of chemotherapy drugs, precautions to prevent pregnancy should be taken throughout treatment with these agents.

Targeted therapies have well-known side effects and toxicities, too. For example, targeting of the epidermal growth factor receptor by cetuximab results in an acneiform rash in most patients. This rash is treated with either topical or systemic antibiotics and is temporary. Some patients can also have severe allergic reactions. Targeting of VEGF by bevacizumab may result in severe bleeding and impaired wound healing, blood clots, and esophageal perforation. Elevated blood pressure and protein in the urine are common but typically simple to control, and they subside once treatment is complete.

In summary, the role of chemotherapy in the treatment of HNSCC has evolved considerably over the past 20 years. The changes have been particularly dramatic among patients with locally or regionally advanced disease, in which chemotherapy figures prominently in the management of unresectable disease, nasopharynx cancer, oropharynx cancer, organ preservation programs, and the poor risk adjuvant setting. Although treatment with chemotherapy certainly carries risks and side effects, there are significant benefits from its use regarding disease control. Close monitoring and management by the treating oncologist minimizes the impact of treatment side effects.

The continued development of new drugs in the fight against HNSCC is critical. Well-done clinical trials are a fundamental part of this process and greatly assist in determining how and when to optimally use chemotherapy to improve disease control outcomes. These studies are often an excellent treatment option for patients and deserve support and participation whenever possible.

References

Adelstein, D. J., Li, Y., Adams, G. L., Wagner, H., Jr., Kish, J. A., Ensley, J. F., et al. (2003). An intergroup phase III comparison of standard radiation therapy and two schedules of concurrent chemoradiotherapy in patients with unresectable squamous cell head and neck cancer. *Journal of Clinical Oncology, 21*, 92–98.

Al-Sarraf, M., LeBlanc, M., Giri, P. G., Fu, K. K., Cooper, J., Vuong, T., et al. (1998). Chemoradiotherapy versus radiotherapy in patients with advanced nasopharyngeal cancer: Phase III randomized intergroup study 0099. *Journal of Clinical Oncology, 16*, 1310–1317.

Bernier, J., Cooper, J. S., Pajak, T. F., van Glabbeke, M., Bourhis, J., Forastiere, A. A., et al. (2005). Defining risk levels in locally advanced head and neck cancers: A comparative analysis of concurrent postoperative radiation plus chemotherapy trials of the EORTC (#22931) and RTOG (#9501). *Head & Neck, 27*, 843–850.

Bernier, J., Domenge, C., Ozsahin, M., Matuszewska, K., Lefebvre, J. L., Greiner, R. H., et al. (2004). Postoperative irradiation with or without concomitant chemotherapy for locally advanced head and neck cancer. *New England Journal of Medicine, 350*, 1945–1952.

Brizel, D. M., Albers, M. E., Fisher, S. R., Scher, R. L., Richtsmeier, W. J., Hars, V., et al. (1998). Hyperfractionated irradiation with or without concurrent chemotherapy for locally advanced head and neck cancer. *New England Journal of Medicine, 338*, 1798–1804.

Brizel, D. M., Wasserman, T. H., Henke, M., Strnad, V., Rudat, V., Monnier, A., et al. (2000). Phase III randomized trial of amifostine as a radioprotector in head and neck cancer. *Journal of Clinical Oncology, 18*, 3339–3345.

Calais, G., Alfonsi, M., Bardet, E., Sire, C., Germain, T., Bergerot, P., et al. (1999). Randomized trial of radiation therapy versus concomitant chemotherapy and radiation therapy for advanced-stage oropharynx carcinoma. *Journal of the National Cancer Institute, 91*, 2081–2086.

Chambers, M. S., Posner, M., Jones, C. U., Biel, M. A., Hodge, K. M., Vitti, R., et al. (2007). Cevimeline for the treatment of postirradiation xerostomia in patients with head and neck cancer. *International Journal of Radiation Oncology, Biology, Physics, 68 (4)*, 1102-1109.

Cohen, E. E., Lingen, M. W., & Vokes, E. E. (2004). The expanding role of systemic therapy in head and neck cancer. *Journal of Clinical Oncology, 22*, 1743–1752.

Cooper, J. S., Pajak, T. F., Forastiere, A. A., Jacobs, J., Campbell, B. H., Saxman, S. B., et al. (2004). Postoperative concurrent radiotherapy and chemotherapy for high-risk squamous-cell carcinoma of the head and neck. *New England Journal of Medicine, 350*, 1937–1944.

Forastiere, A. A., Maor, M., Weber, R., Pajak, T., Glisson, B., Trotti, A., et al. (2006). Long-term results of intergroup RTOG 91-11: A phase III trial to preserve the larynx—Induction cisplatin/5FU and radiation therapy versus concurrent cisplatin and radiation therapy versus radiation therapy. *Journal of Clinical Oncology, 24*, Abstract 5517.

Fountzilas, G., Ciuleanu, E., Dafni, U., Plataniotis, G., Kalogera-Fountzila, A., Samantas, E., et al. (2004). Concomitant radiochemotherapy vs radiotherapy alone in patients with head and neck cancer: A Hellenic Cooperative Oncology Group phase III study. *Medical Oncology, 21*, 95–107.

Henke, M., Laszig, R., Rube, C., Schafer, U., Haase, K. D., Schilcher, B., et al. (2003). Erythropoietin to treat head and neck cancer patients with anaemia undergoing radiotherapy: Randomised, double-blind, placebo-controlled trial. *Lancet, 362*(9392), 1255–1260.

Hitt, R., Lopez-Pousa, A., Martinez-Trufero, J., Escrig, V., Carles, J., Rizo, A., et al. (2005). Phase III study comparing cisplatin plus fluorouracil to paclitaxel, cisplatin, and fluorouracil induction chemotherapy followed by chemoradiotherapy in locally advanced head and neck cancer. *Journal of Clinical Oncology, 23*, 8636–8645.

Johnson, J. T., Ferretti, G. A., Nethery, W. J., Valdez, I. H., Fox, P. C., Ng, D., et al. (1993). Oral pilocarpine for post-irradiation xerostomia in patients with head and neck cancer. *New England Journal of Medicine, 329*, 390–395.

Leon, X., Hitt, R., Constenla, M., Rocca, A., Stupp, R., Kovacs, A. F., et al. (2005). A retrospective analysis of the outcome of patients with recurrent and/or metastatic squamous cell carcinoma of the head and neck refractory to a platinum-based chemotherapy. *Clinical Oncology (Royal College of Radiologists), 17*, 418–424.

Pignon, J. P., Bourhis, J., Domenge, C., & Designe, L. (2000). Chemotherapy added to locoregional treatment for head and neck squamous-cell carcinoma: Three meta-analyses of updated individual data. MACH-NC Collaborative Group. Meta-analysis of chemotherapy on head and neck cancer. *Lancet, 355*, 949–955.

Posner, M. R., Hershock, D. M., Blajman, C. R., Mickiewicz, E., Winquist, E., Gorbounova, E., et al. (2007). Cisplatin and fluorouracil alone or with docetaxel in head and neck cancer. *New England Journal of Medicine*, *357*, 1705-1715.

Shah, K., Lincoff, A. M., & Young, J. B. (1996). Anthracycline-induced cardiotoxicity. *Annals of Internal Medicine*, *125*(1), 47–58.

Vermorken, J., Mesia, R., Vega, V., Remenar, E., Hitt, R., Kawecki, A., et al. (2007). Cetuximab extends survival of patients with recurrent or metastatic SCCHN when added to first line platinum therapy—Results of a randomized phase III (Extreme) study. *Journal of Clinical Oncology*, *25*(18S), Abstract No. 6091.

Vermorken, J. B., Remenar, E., van Herpen, C., Gorlia, T., Mesia, R., Degardin, M., et al. (2007). Cisplatin, Fluorouracil, and Docetaxel in Unresectable Head and Neck Cancer. *New England Journal of Medicine*, *357*, 1695-1704.

5

MEETING THE CHALLENGES OF GOOD ORAL CARE IN THE MANAGEMENT OF HEAD AND NECK CANCER

James J. Sciubba, DMD, PhD

The management of oral and head and neck cancer almost always produces a series of side effects that range from the merely bothersome to some that can be severely debilitating and affect overall cancer management and quality of life. Often there is the immediate need to begin treatment without mention or discussion of specific side effects that each patient may be facing. These could be related to the surgical management as a stand-alone treatment or to surgery in combination with radiation therapy and/or chemotherapy. The increasing use of chemotherapy in certain forms of head and neck cancer carries its own set of possible adverse effects.

The oral complications or side effects of head and neck cancer management vary widely from patient to patient and according to the treatment rendered, ranging from mild and temporary to severe and long lasting, even lifelong in many cases. With this in mind, the routine management of the mouth and the teeth becomes an important issue, with the patient's dental care provider being a critical member of the management team along with the cancer surgeon, radiation oncologist, medical oncologist, speech and swallowing therapists, and others. In cases in which surgically created anatomical deficits are present, a maxillofacial prosthodontist will also be involved.

Surgical Management

When surgery alone is the treatment rendered for relatively limited or stage I and II cancers, posttreatment dental and oral management may be almost routine in nature. When a surgically created deficit may result in speech alteration, the patient may require the services of a trained speech pathologist. When a swallowing deficit or difficulty is encountered, specialized tests may be needed to identify the specific reason for the dysfunction with swallowing therapy to follow, along with a modified diet until the results of therapy will permit the patient to consume a wider range of foods.

When removal of a portion of the upper or lower jaw is a component of the surgical management, reconstruction becomes an issue. This complex area of care often relies on coordination of several providers, including the cancer surgeon, the reconstructive surgeon, and the maxillofacial prosthodontist. The collective goal is the restoration of function and aesthetics of the jaws and the oro-facial complex. This may be achieved with the use of specialized oral appliances such as an obturator. This prosthesis is designed to seal off the surgically created upper jaw and palatal defects from the mouth, allowing normal chewing, swallowing, and speech as well as improving aesthetic appearance. Obturators may be retained or held in place and stabilized by the use of dental implants or may be retained by modification of existing natural teeth if there are adequate numbers remaining in the upper jaw after surgery.

The reconstructive surgeon may also choose to do a bone graft to correct a surgical defect. This procedure involves the harvesting of a portion of bone and muscle with its own blood supply from either the leg or arm and transferring it to the surgically created defect in the oral and neck area. The artery and vein of the graft are then joined with an artery and vein in the neck so that the graft survives and functions. Subsequent to healing, dental implants will be placed into the grafted bone by an oral and maxillofacial surgeon. Following integration or fusion of the implant to the bone, the maxillofacial prosthodontist will then be able to construct dental bridgework or a removable appliance over the implants where stability and excellent function will be afforded.

Radiation Therapy

Dental input and intervention as it concerns the delivery of radiation therapy is of great importance and is ideally established when the decision is made to undergo this option of treatment. Most radiation oncologists integrate the dental component of care on a routine basis, referring the cancer patient for a dental evaluation prior to initiating radiation therapy. Necessary extractions are performed, allowing early healing in advance of radiation therapy.

Once the dental evaluation is completed and radiation treatment is under way, a rigorous oral care prevention regimen must be developed. The dentist should carefully explain to the patient the importance of this lifelong regimen as it relates to the side effects of radiation therapy and its long-term effects. The patient should be aware of the early side effects of head and neck radiation therapy, which are likely to include radiation-induced dry mouth (xerostomia) and mouth and throat soreness (mucositis). The imminent reduction of saliva flow following standard radiation delivery techniques may likely produce several functional problems, including difficulty in eating and swallowing and some alterations in speech.

As a result of the dry mouth, the twice-daily application of high-strength fluoride becomes mandatory in an effort to prevent the rapid onset of dental decay associated with dryness. This application can be accomplished by the use of a tray appliance or mouth guard into which fluoride gel is placed. Alternatively, some practitioners prefer to use the same form of fluoride gel on the toothbrush instead of toothpaste on a twice-daily basis. Neutral sodium fluoride, 5,000 parts per million, or stannous fluoride 0.4% are recommended and should be discussed with the dentist or dental hygienist. In addition, over-the-counter fluoride rinses are available and are often recommended to supplement high-strength fluoride gels.

When using trays or "mouth guard appliances," a thin layer of fluoride is placed into the tray and placed over the teeth for 10 minutes. The patient should avoid swallowing excess fluoride. After the trays are removed, they should be washed under cold water and stored in a cool, well-ventilated place. It is recommended that the patient not eat or rinse for 30 minutes after the trays are removed.

To combat the problem of reduction or absence of saliva, two commonly prescribed drugs are available—cevimeline (Evoxac®) and pilocarpine (Salagen®). Stimulation of saliva with sugar-free candy or chewing gum is often helpful, as are saliva substitutes in the form of sprays and gels. Over time some return of saliva production may be noticed but rarely to preradiation levels.

An aggressive and necessary dental prevention program is important to avoid the need for dental extractions in the years to come due to decay or periodontal (gum) disease. If an oral surgical procedure is necessary, there is a significant risk of developing a condition known as osteoradionecrosis (bone death due to radiation). This condition, resulting from a reduction of blood flow within the jaw secondary to radiation therapy, is permanent. As a result of less blood flow to the jaw, any tooth extraction site may not heal properly and may become infected, thus characterizing osteoradionecrosis. Management of this complication may include administration of hyperbaric oxygen therapy before and after a planned extraction in an effort to increase the number of new blood vessels in the area, thus promoting healing without infection and without bone becoming necrotic or dying. If osteonecrosis develops, a similar treatment with hyperbaric oxygen precedes removal of dead bone, followed again with a second course of hyperbaric treatment.

While most dental providers are aware of cancer treatment and the effects of radiation therapy on the mouth, salivary glands, and the teeth, some might not know how to manage the complications. If this is the case, most radiation oncologists and head and neck surgeons should be able to assist the patient with a proper dental referral.

Other radiation-induced oral complications include altered, diminished, or loss of taste sensation and radiation-induced mucositis or mouth and throat sores. While little can be done about taste alterations, there is often a return of this sense in the months following treatment. Treatment for mucositis may include salt water and baking soda rinses; topical anesthetics; or rinses containing combinations of a topical anesthetic, a soothing liquid such as milk of magnesia, and a flavoring agent. Several commercially available or over-the-counter nonalcoholic mouth rinses may also be helpful (Oasis, Crest Pro-Health, Biotene). Chapter 11 contains a comprehensive product listing.

During the early phases of radiation therapy, actual dental treatment short of tooth extractions and bony periodontal surgery can proceed normally. Routine cleanings (prophylaxis procedures), fillings, bridgework, and removable dentures are permissible without any increased level of precautions.

The issue of dental implant placement in the irradiated jaw following a strict protocol that may include hyperbaric oxygen therapy has been studied. The necessity of this adjunct remains controversial; however, good long-term results have been achieved using such implants. Implants may also be placed in bone grafts with similar functional results as previously discussed.

Maintenance of oral moisture is often a problem, in particular when radiation therapy includes the salivary glands within the treatment field. Patients may need to modify their diet with the addition of softer or blended foods until salivary function improves. Small bites of food that are lukewarm or cool and avoidance of abrasive and highly spiced foods are often necessary. Special cookbooks are available for the oral and head and neck cancer patient that suggest a wide range of foods and recipes that are more tolerable and nutritionally sound. If eating a normal or modified diet is not yet possible, calorie and protein intake can be achieved with liquid products such as Boost, Ensure, Scandishake, and others. Lubricants such as aloe vera or lanolin on the lips may be helpful.

Some consideration may be given to the use of remineralizing solutions to help stop the process of calcium loss from the teeth in areas of very early decay. Patients will be susceptible to dental decay at a much higher level than before treatment as a result of mouth dryness and the loss of the protective substances that saliva contains; therefore, patients should visit the dentist more often than before treatment. As an extension of the prevention strategy, consideration must be given to performing dental procedures as early as possible.

Chemotherapy

The emerging role of chemotherapy in the management of oral and head neck cancer has heightened the risk of treatment-induced mucositis. While the mechanism of mucositis production differs from that due to radiation therapy, the result is essentially the same and will be considered collectively. This side effect can be heightened or amplified when radiation therapy is also a component of overall management.

Severe mucositis can be present in upwards of 90% of head and neck cancer patients receiving chemoradiotherapy, thus imposing an additional burden on quality of life and resources. Management of this problem remains difficult, with several agents now in clinical trial. The traditional approaches with topical lidocaine and orally administered analgesics, including opioids for pain, are only marginally effective as are salt water/bicarbonate rinses. Recent preliminary studies showed that low-energy laser therapy reduced symptoms dramatically. Additionally, studies employing the use of the growth factors palifermin and velifermin have shown great promise, in particular when considered in a combined manner with laser treatment. Final recommendations await the completion of further clinical studies concerning these modalities.

Posttreatment Care

Maintenance of teeth, jawbone integrity, and dental appliances becomes a lifelong consideration. Preventing infection of the supporting oral structures and gum tissues and maintaining tooth integrity and overall dental health are crucial. To help accomplish this, dental care will likely be more extensive than it was before cancer treatment started, including more frequent visits for routine follow-up and maintenance with the dentist, dental hygienist, and prosthodontist.

Patients should inform any new dental provider not familiar with their cancer diagnosis and treatment that they have had chemotherapy or radiation therapy. This may result in adjustment of care and formulation of a treatment plan that will include a more aggressive preventive strategy and increased follow-up visits.

By far the most important aspect of dental health preservation, dental restorations, and appliance longevity is faithful adherence to home care measures. These measures include careful use of dental floss before brushing and use of fluoride-containing toothpaste or dental trays as stated earlier. Use of regular toothpaste without whiteners and tartar control formulation is encouraged. If brushing after meals is not possible, patients should rinse with water, avoiding use of excessively flavored or "spicy" flavors such as those containing cinnamon or cinnamon flavoring that may cause burning of the mouth lining.

In summary, the adherence to rigorous dental and oral care and responsible dietary habits during and following cancer treatment is essential. Early communication with the entire management team and required follow-up care on a routine basis will help ensure oral health and maintenance of function into the future.

Further Reading

Chambers, M. S., Garden, A. S., Kies, M. S., & Martin, J. W. (2004). Radiation-induced xerostomia in patients with head and neck cancer: Pathogenesis, impact on quality of life, and management. *Head & Neck, 26*, 796–807.

Chiapasco, M., Biglioli, F., Autelitano, L., Romeo, E., & Brusati, R. (2006). Clinical outcome of dental implants placed in fibula-free flaps for the reconstruction of maxillo-mandibular defects following ablation for tumors or osteoradionecrosis. *Clinical Oral Implants Research, 17*, 220–228.

Donoff, R. B. (2006). Treatment of the irradiated patient with dental implants: The case against hyperbaric oxygen treatment. *Journal of Oral and Maxillofacial Surgery, 64*, 819–822.

Duke, R. L., Campbell, B. H., Indresano, A. T., Eaton, D. J., Marbella, A. M., Myers, K. B., et al. (2005). Dental status and quality of life in long-term head and neck cancer survivors. *Laryngoscope, 115*, 678–683.

Granstrom, G. (2006). Placement of dental implants in irradiated bone: The case for using hyperbaric oxygen. *Journal of Oral and Maxillofacial Surgery, 64*, 812–818.

Kielbassa, A. M., Hinkelbein, W., Hellwig, E., & Meyer-Lackel, H. (2006). Radiation-related damage to dentition. *Lancet Oncology, 7*, 326–335.

Miller, E. H., & Quinn, A. I. (2006). Dental considerations in the management of head and neck cancer patients. *Otolaryngologic Clinics of North America, 39*, 319–332.

Omer, O., MacCarthy, D., Nunn, J., & Cotter, E. (2005). Oral health needs of the head and neck radiotherapy patient: 2. Oral and dental care before, during and after radiotherapy. *Dental Update, 32*, 575-576, 578-580, 582.

Peled, M., El-Naaj, I. A., Lipin, Y., & Ardekian, L. (2005). The use of free fibular flap for functional mandibular reconstruction. *Journal of Oral and Maxillofacial Surgery, 63*, 220-224.

6

MEETING THE CHALLENGES OF TARGETED THERAPY AND SKIN CARE

Mario E. Lacouture, MD

Cancer Treatments and the Skin

Anticancer treatments such as chemotherapy and radiation owe their effectiveness to an interference with rapidly growing cells (a hallmark of cancer). This explains the frequent occurrence of side effects in normal tissues that are also composed of rapidly growing cells, such as the skin, hair, and nails. In particular, the newly introduced targeted therapies result in distinctive dermatological side effects that may affect quality of life and in some cases result in treatment interruption or discontinuation. Interestingly, these new targeted therapies are directed at specific receptor molecules of cancer and may produce fewer side effects than conventional chemotherapy; which makes the significance of dermatological events resulting from targeted therapies greatly heightened (Robert et al., 2005).

Improvements in chemotherapy and radiation have allowed for more precise "targeting" of tumor cells, resulting in minimal or no side effects to the blood and internal organs. This has allowed for better clinical responses leading to longer survival. Treatments that are "targeted" offer the promise of a more favorable safety profile. This is partly a result of their ability to affect molecules that are pivotal in cancer cells. Coincidentally, one of the primary receptor molecules involved in head and neck squamous cell carcinoma (HNSCC) is known as the epidermal growth factor receptor (EGFR). This receptor is targeted by cetuximab (Erbitux®), which has been approved by the U.S. Food and Drug Administration (FDA) for the treatment of HNSCC in combination with radiation (http://www.fda.gov).

The skin is composed of three major layers: the epidermis (outermost layer), which is composed of rapidly growing cells; the underlying layer (dermis), which contains nerves, blood vessels, and hairs and provides structural support; and the deeper fatty layer (or hypodermis), which protects against cold temperature and trauma. Thus, the close proximity and similarity of the skin to tissues affected by HNSCC make it a categorical "innocent bystander" subject to the effects of radiation therapy and targeted anticancer drugs. Efforts to reduce the impact of cancer treatments on the skin should be implemented early. Patients' knowledge of side effects and their early reporting to the oncology team will help to ensure that consistent anticancer treatment and quality of life are maintained and that the maximum benefit from therapy is gained.

Targeted Anticancer Treatments and the Skin

The EGFR is required for normal skin, hair, and nail growth and overall health (King et al, 1990). Consequently, when its activity is blocked, cells are unable to function properly, resulting in skin inflammation, abnormal growth, tenderness, or itching and raising the possibility of infection (Lacouture, 2006). The potentially serious dermatological side effects resulting from targeted therapies may impact the treatment of HNSCC as they may lead to modification of the use of the anticancer treatment drug as reported in 17% of patients or its permanent discontinuation in approximately 4% of patients (Bonner et al., 2006).

Drugs targeting the EGFR have also been approved in other tumors, such as colorectal, lung, and pancreatic cancers. Considerable information has been collected on the appearance and management of dermatological side effects in these other settings. Whereas these observations may give some insight into the development of side effects in patients with HNSCC, they must not be applied directly in this setting for two reasons. First, in HNSCC, EGFR-targeting drugs, when given with radiation therapy, are usually used for a short period of time (approximately 8 weeks) whereas in other cancers, when given alone, they are used indefinitely, creating a new set of side effects (Roe et al., 2006). Second, the sequence in which radiation therapy is administered to head and neck cancer patients also affects the way in which the side effects appear in the skin. Thus, radiation therapy given prior to a targeted therapy will result in the sparing of EGFR-targeting drug-induced rash, and radiation therapy given concurrently with drug therapy will result in the worsening of rash in the radiated areas such as the neck.

Side Effects of Treatment on Skin

The most frequent and clinically significant side effects from the use of EGFR-targeting drugs occur in the skin. A rash affecting the face, scalp, and upper trunk will appear in as many as 87% of patients receiving cetuximab (Erbitux®) and may be associated with itching or tenderness. The majority of these cases are mild to moderate, but as many as 17% of cases may be severe and require the modification of the drug due to discomfort and possible skin infection. It is noteworthy that although the rash may look like acne, for which it has been incorrectly labeled "acneiform," it is not acne and does not respond to most topical acne medications.

The rash appears within the first few weeks after the first infusion of the drug and is characterized by several phases (Lacouture, 2006). In the first, occurring within the initial days, a sensation of sunburn with swelling of the nose predominates. If prophylactic treatment against rash has not already taken place, it is advisable to inform the oncologist or oncology nurse so that treatment can be initiated to prevent progression to a more severe grade. In the next phase, which occurs at the end of the 1st week or beginning of the 2nd week, red-yellow bumps appear on the skin, which may bleed and itch. Overall the size and number of bumps tend to peak in the 2nd to 3rd week, then slowly decrease in severity, but may still require treatment. These bumps are not indicative of infection and will not be spread to other people. At the end of the 3rd or 4th weeks, a crust forms in the areas where the bumps are located. Finally, after the rash has resolved, redness of the face ensues, leaving some areas with dilated blood vessels.

An important correlation has been observed in which those patients who develop a very bad rash have a better response in terms of the cancer and longer survival (Perez-Soler & Saltz, 2005). This remarkable connection underscores the notion that people that develop rash should be maintained on EGFR-inhibitor treatment because they are the ones that could benefit the most. Notwithstanding this fact, those who do not develop rash should not be discouraged, as excellent responses have also been observed in the absence of the rash.

Other skin side effects that appear after the 2nd to 4th week include dry and itchy skin. This side effect has been reported in 15% of those patients treated, with 30% of these patients reporting dry and itchy skin of the fingertips and heels of the feet, resulting in paper-cut fissures causing tenderness and stinging (Roe et al., 2006).

Side Effects on Hair

Hair loss, as seen with conventional chemotherapy, is not characteristic of EGFR-targeting drugs. However, hair loss can develop in as many as 4% of patients and tends to occur after 4 to 6 months of continuous EGFR-targeted treatment. It usually affects only the front of the scalp (as seen in older men). On the other hand, the rash that occurs on the face in the first few weeks can extend beyond the face and upper trunk and may involve the scalp, leading to itchy bumps along with hair loss. Exceptional growth of eyelashes and facial hair has been observed in 6% of treated patients (Robert et al., 2005). The texture of the hair may also change, appearing more brittle and curlier as time goes on. Overall, hair problems may appear several months after treatment and are not likely to occur in the 2 month course of HNSCC therapy.

Side Effects on Nails

After the 6th week of treatment, inflammation and redness around the fingernails and toenails occur in about 40% of patients (Roe et al., 2006). This inflammation around the nails is known as paronychia and may impair the ability to perform daily activities, such as grooming, buttoning clothes, or handling objects because of the associated tenderness. It is very important that the health care team be informed at the first sign of this effect (redness, tenderness, or fraying of the cuticles). Brittle nails may also appear, although infrequently.

Radiation Therapy and the Skin

Despite remarkable advances in radiation oncology, radiodermatitis (skin inflammation, with redness, swelling, and pain) remains a common side effect of radiation therapy. In the study that led to the FDA's approval of treatment using cetuximab combined with radiotherapy, 86% of patients receiving combined treatment suffered from radiodermatitis, of which 23% of the cases were considered severe (Bonner et al., 2006). Notably, in the absence of cetuximab, this side effect was seen in a similar number of patients treated with radiation alone. However, anecdotal reports (Budach et al, 2007) and clinical experience at a large-volume referral center, the SERIES (Skin and Eye Reactions to Inhibitors of EGFR and kinaseS) Clinic (Lacouture, Basti, Patel, & Benson, 2006) at Northwestern University in Chicago, suggests that combining EGFR-inhibitor and radiation therapy may lead to more severe radiodermatitis (Lacouture, Hwang, Marymont, & Patel, 2007). More studies are needed to confirm this observation, and this should be set in the context that this combination led to significantly greater anticancer activity than either therapy alone. A paradoxical finding is that patients who receive radiation therapy more than 3 months prior to EGFR-inhibitor drug often have less rash and radiodermatitis (Bossi et al., 2007).

Prevention and Treatment of Dermatological Side Effects

There are two key elements that help to minimize the impact of dermatological side effects on quality of life: (a) early recognition of the side effects so that prompt treatments can be instituted and (b) the use of treatments tailored to the location and type of side effect. A proactive approach dictates that therapy begin even before the onset of anticancer treatment so that the chances of development and severity are minimal. This is an approach that has already shown promise in the treatment of rash to EGFR-inhibitor drugs. Knowledge of the sequence of side effect development is critical to anticipating these dermatological side effects: rash (weeks 1 to 3), nail inflammation (weeks 2 to 6), dry skin (weeks 6 to 8), and hair problems (weeks 12 to 24) (Lynch et al., 2007).

Several measures can be initiated prior to or when therapy is started:

- Use of a broad-spectrum sunscreen (containing zinc oxide or titanium dioxide) with an SPF (sun protection factor) of at least 15
- Use of mild soaps for showering or bathing (Dove®, Cetaphil®, Basis®)
- Use of detergents that are free of fragrances or perfumes (All® free clear , Tide® free)
- Use of lukewarm instead of hot water in the shower or bath
- Use of moisturizers containing ammonium lactate (Am-Lactin®) or 10% urea daily, especially on very dry areas of the hands and feet
- Avoidance of sun exposure, and wearing a broad-brimmed hat
- The possibility of prophylactic therapy with prescription creams or oral tetracycline antibiotics
- Avoidance of tight-fitting shoes or trauma around the nails
- Having contact information of the oncologist or oncology nurse available in the event they are needed

If the rash develops, the doctor may prescribe a corticosteroid or antibiotic cream, which is to be applied thinly and evenly on the face, chest and upper back, or other affected areas. If the scalp is affected, the dermatologist may suggest foams or shampoos containing corticosteroids. Corticosteroids work by blocking inflammation, a key element in rash formation, itching, and tenderness. In some cases oral antibiotics may be prescribed in order to reduce the severity of the rash, which should be taken on a daily basis (Scope et al, 2007).

Treatment of rash has been shown to lead to more complete improvement when it is mild in severity, so informing the doctor at this mild stage is important to achieve good results. The same principle is applied for radiodermatitis; studies have shown that prophylactic treatment with topical steroids minimizes the severity and discomfort associated with this reaction (Bostrom, Lindman,

Swartling, Berne, & Bergh, 2001). Keep in mind, however, that although it is safe to use topical steroid creams for radiodermatitis, these should be wiped off before the radiation therapy is administered to minimize augmentation of the energy in those areas.

As discussed previously, nail inflammation is not common in patients with HNSCC. If redness, pain, or swelling occurs despite adequate moisturization as indicated earlier, it is important to avoid infection. Soaking the tips of fingers or toes in a solution of white vinegar diluted 1:10 in water provides antiseptic relief. If drainage from areas around the nail occurs, oral antibiotic therapy may be needed (Fox, 2007). For severely dry skin, the doctor may prescribe exfoliants to remove flaking and scaling skin (e.g. ammonium lactate 12% creams). Always try creams on a small (quarter-size) area of skin so that if irritation occurs, it is not as severe. For itching, use a cream that is also anti-itch (Sarna Ultra® cream). For more severe itching, Regenecare® gel is a good option but should be limited to smaller areas because it contains the anesthetic lidocaine. Patients with itching report immediate relief by keeping these creams in the refrigerator because they provide an immediate cooling effect when applied. Sometimes, oral medicines against itching may be needed, such as antihistamines and pregabalin (Lyrica®), which may cause drowsiness, so taking them at night will provide a better night's sleep (Porzio, Aielli, Verna, Porto, Tudini, et al., 2006).

In the great majority of cases, dermatological side effects from radiation therapy and novel targeted drugs will not lead to long-term sequelae, and anticancer treatments will not need to be modified. This can be achieved by following several principles—employing preventive measures and initiating treatments to offset side effects as early as possible. By playing an active role in treatment, patients will be able to get the most benefit from therapy and maintain an optimal sense of well-being.

References

Erbitux approval summary. Retrieved July 15, 2007, from www.fda.gov

Bonner, J. A., Harari, P. M., Giralt, J., Azarnia, N., Shin, D. M., Cohen, R. B., et al. (2006). Radiotherapy plus cetuximab for squamous-cell carcinoma of the head and neck. *New England Journal of Medicine, 354,* 567–578.

Bossi, P., Liberatoscioli, C., Bergamini, C., Locati, L., Fava, S., Rinaldi, G., et al. (2007). Previously irradiated areas spared from skin toxicity induced by cetuximab in six patients: Implications for the administration of EGFR inhibitors in previously irradiated patients. *Annals of Oncology, 18,* 601–602.

Bostrom, A., Lindman, H., Swartling, C., Berne, B., & Bergh, J. (2001). Potent corticosteroid cream (mometasone furoate) significantly reduces acute radiation dermatitis: Results from a double-blind, randomized study. *Radiotherapy & Oncology, 59,* 257–265.

Budach, W., Bölke, E., & Homey, B. (2007). Severe cutaneous reaction during radiation therapy with concurrent cetuximab. *New England Journal of Medicine, 357*(5), 514–515.

Fox, L. P. (2007). Nail toxicity associated with epidermal growth factor receptor inhibitor therapy. *Journal of the American Academy of Dermatology, 56*(3), 460–465.

King, L. E., Jr., Gates, R. E., Stoscheck, C. M., & Nanney, L. B. (1990). The EGF/TGF alpha receptor in skin. *Journal of Investigative Dermatology, 94*(Suppl. 6), 164S–170S.

Lacouture, M. E. (2006). Mechanisms of cutaneous toxicities to EGFR inhibitors. *Nature Reviews Cancer, 6,* 803–812.

Lacouture, M. E., Basti, S., Patel, J., & Benson, A., 3rd. (2006). The SERIES clinic: An interdisciplinary approach to the management of toxicities of EGFR inhibitors. *Journal of Supportive Oncology, 4,* 236–238.

Lacouture, M. E., Hwang, C., Marymont, M. H., & Patel, J. (2007). Temporal dependence of the effect of radiation on erlotinib-induced skin rash. *Journal of Clinical Oncology, 25,* 2140.

Lynch, T. J., Kim, E. S., Eaby, B., Garey, J., West, D. P., & Lacouture M. E. (2007, May). Epidermal growth factor receptor inhibitor-associated cutaneous toxicities: An evolving paradigm in clinical management. *Oncologist, 12*(5), 610–621.

Perez-Soler, R., & Saltz, L. (2005). Cutaneous adverse effects with HER1/EGFR-targeted agents: Is there a silver lining? *Journal of Clinical Oncology, 23,* 5235–5246.

Porzio, G., Aielli, F., Verna, L., Porto, C., Tudini, M., Cannita, K., et al. (2006). Efficacy of pregabalin in the management of cetuximab-related itch. *Journal of Pain and Symptom Management, 32,* 397–398.

Robert, C., Soria, J. C., Spatz, A., Le Cesne, A., Malka, D., Pautier, P., et al. (2005). Cutaneous side-effects of kinase inhibitors and blocking antibodies. *Lancet Oncology, 6,* 491–500.

Roe, E., Garcia Muret, M. P., Marcuello, E., Capdevila, J., Pallares, C., & Alomar, A. (2006). Description and management of cutaneous side effects during cetuximab or erlotinib treatments: A prospective study of 30 patients. *Journal of the American Academy of Dermatology, 55,* 429–437.

Scope, A., Agero, A. L., Dusza, S. W., Myskowski, P. L., Lieb, J. A., Saltz, L., et al. (2007). Randomized double-blind trial of prophylactic oral minocycline and topical tazarotene for cetuximab-associated acne-like eruption. *Journal of Clinical Oncology, 25*(34), 5390–5396.

7

MEETING THE CHALLENGES OF COMMUNICATION AND SWALLOWING DISORDERS AND TREATMENT IN HEAD AND NECK CANCER

Bonnie Martin-Harris, PhD
Julie Blair, MA, CCC-SLP

The processes of speaking and swallowing require little thought or effort for most healthy adults. However, the underlying complexities of these processes become evident following head and neck cancer treatments that often involve structural and functional alterations to the mouth, throat, and esophagus. Much of what has been learned about speech and swallowing function, disorders, and treatments stems from experiences gained from patients who have undergone treatments to the head and neck. Though cancer treatments and rehabilitation efforts have undergone marked advances, persistent speech and swallowing dysfunction of varying degrees continues to be a major problem for many head and neck cancer survivors.

Communication

Verbal communication is reliant on multiple interdependent subsystems. These include respiration (breathing), phonation (voicing), resonance (timbre), and articulation (speech). Disruption of any one of these subsystems related to a disease process, surgical alteration, or other intervention may result in altered oral communication ability (Casper & Colton, 1998; Sullivan & Guilford, 1999; Ward & van As-Brooks, 2007).

Respiration is the driving force behind voice production. Respiratory function for voice and speech production may be impaired in a variety of ways. Patients with head and neck cancer may have a coexisting pulmonary disease such as emphysema or chronic obstructive pulmonary disease (COPD) that increases the respiratory effort associated with talking. Respiration for speech production is also disrupted by the presence of a tracheostomy tube because much of the lung air is redirected from the larynx to the front of the neck to ease patients' breathing. The vocal folds cannot vibrate as efficiently without the full force of airflow from below, and a breathy, weak, or hoarse voice may result. Special tracheostomy valves may be placed over the opening of the tube to assist patients with directing lung air back through the larynx, thereby improving the quality and volume of the voice (Dikeman & Kazandjian, 2003; Stemple, Glaze, & Gerderman, 2000; Sullivan & Guilford, 1999; Ward & van As-Brooks, 2007).

Phonation is the process of voice production that relies on vibration of the vocal folds (vocal cords) housed in the larynx (voice box). Voice quality, pitch, and loudness may be altered if the cancer surgery or radiation treatment involves the larynx or if the patient has a swallowing problem and is unable to clear the throat after each swallow gesture. An alternative sound source, such as an artificial larynx or special speaking valve, may be recommended in some cases when removal of the larynx is required (Casper & Colton, 1998; Stemple, Glaze, & Gerderman, 2000; Sullivan & Guilford, 1999; Ward & van As-Brooks, 2007).

Resonance is the effect on the voice related to the shape of the throat, mouth, and nasal cavities. This shaping of the sound gives rise to the timbre and richness of sound produced by the larynx. Alterations made to the shape or contours of the vocal tract following surgery to the head and neck may result in changes to the patient's and listener's perception of the voice (Casper & Colton, 1998; Stemple, Glaze, & Gerderman, 2000).

Articulation is the process through which the sounds are formed by contact of the articulators, which include the tongue, teeth, palate, and lips. Approximation or full contact of these structures with one another results in the characteristic sounds used during speech production. Each sound is defined by its manner and placement. The manner refers to how the sound and air are shaped. Some sounds stop the flow of air, releasing it in a burst ("t") whereas others shape the sound into a directed ("s") stream. Placement refers to where the sound is made, for example, between the lips ("p"), tongue to teeth ("th"), and tongue to palate ("k"). Alterations to the structure or mobility of the articulators will disrupt the precision of the sounds. Restricted movement of the upper (maxilla) and lower (mandible) jaw occurs in some patients following surgeries and radiation treatment to the oral cavity. This condition is referred to as *trismus*, and it may interfere with articulation and resonance as well as mouth opening for efficient eating and drinking (Casper & Colton, 1998; Sullivan & Guilford, 1999; Ward & van As-Brooks, 2007).

Treatment of the head and neck cancer through radiation, chemotherapy, or surgery may result in altered integrity, shape, and mobility of the structures involved in speech and voice production. In addition to influencing oral communication ability, these changes may also have a negative impact on swallowing function (Logemann, 1998; Sullivan & Guilford, 1999; Ward & van As-Brooks, 2007) .

Swallowing

Swallowing function is highly dependent on smooth and coordinated movements of the structures of the oral cavity, pharynx (throat), larynx, and esophagus (tube that moves food from the lower throat to the stomach). Swallowing is a complex process in which food and liquid are prepared and transferred from the oral cavity to the stomach. This includes mixing the food with saliva, chewing, pushing the bolus (food or liquid) through the mouth by way of upward and backward motion of the tongue, and lifting of the palate to prevent entry of the bolus into the back of the nose.

Breathing usually stops well before or at least by the time the bolus reaches the back of the mouth. The bolus is then pushed through the pharynx as the larynx closes to protect the trachea and lungs from aspiration (entry of food or liquid below the larynx). Swallowing also includes a brisk upward and forward movement of the larynx that not only aids in closing its valves (including the vocal cords and epiglottis) but also serves to pull open the upper part of the esophagus. There are two valves of the esophagus, one upper and one lower. They are referred to as the upper esophageal sphincter and lower esophageal sphincter. Both sphincters remain tightly closed at rest and open only to allow passage of food or liquid during swallowing, or gas as in the case of belching.

All of this dynamic activity occurs rapidly and within seconds in normal circumstances. However, following surgery, radiation, or chemoradiation, the structures involved in swallowing may move more slowly and less effectively, causing discoordination and effort associated with eating and drinking (Lazarus, 2000; Pauloski, Rademaker, Logemann, 1998; Sullivan & Guilford, 1999; Ward & van As-Brooks, 2007).

Swallowing Disorders

Treatment of head and neck cancer may result in a swallowing disorder (dysphagia) depending on the nature and extent of the cancer treatment. Structures and their associated function may be modified by the size of the tumor, the nature of the surgical resection, and type of reconstruction.

Altered sensation may interfere with airway protection if the patient is unable to feel food or liquid that misdirects into the airway. Radiation and chemotherapy treatments may contribute to alterations in sensation and comfort during swallowing because of acute inflammation, or swelling of the lining of the mouth and throat may occur. Radiation treatment may also alter the function of the salivary glands, resulting in increased thickness of secretions in the mouth and throat. Further, radiation often contributes to a dry mouth and throat (xerostomia), which changes the ease and pleasure associated with chewing and swallowing. Other changes to head and neck tissues associated with radiation treatment, such as fibrosis, often result in stiffening of the mobile structures in the mouth and throat and therefore reduce their range of movement (Sullivan & Guilford, 1999; Lazarus, 2000; Logemann, 1998; Logemann, Pauloski, Rademaker, et al. 1997; Pauloski, Rademaker, Logemann, 1998; Ward & van As-Brooks, 2007).

Advances in the type and delivery of radiation treatment are beginning to demonstrate some easing of these side effects. The acute swallowing problems associated with head and neck treatments are typically temporary and do improve over time and with appropriate speech and swallowing treatment. Swallowing difficulty may persist in some patients, however, long after the initial cancer treatment. The nature of the swallowing treatment plan is driven by appropriate selection and implementation of standardized swallowing assessments with unique tailoring for each individual patient (Logemann, 1998; Sullivan & Guilford, 1999; Ward & van As-Brooks, 2007).

Speech and Swallowing Evaluation

Patients undergoing treatment for head and neck cancer should be seen for consultation by a speech-language pathologist whenever possible prior to initiation of their treatment. This initial visit is an opportunity to establish the patient's baseline communication function, educate the patient and caregivers regarding communication and swallowing rehabilitative options following treatment, and in some cases initiate therapy even prior to beginning treatment. Interaction among the head and neck cancer team is critical to maximize the recovery potential and to ensure continuity of patient care. Members of the specialty team may include some or all of the following, and their respective roles are detailed in other portions of this text: otolaryngologist, nurse, speech-language pathologist, maxillofacial prosthodontist, radiologist, oncologist, gastroenterologist, and physical and occupational therapist. The team creates a diagnostic and treatment plan that follows a protocol dictated not only by the cancer but also by the nature of the speech and swallowing problems and the individual needs of each patient.

There are several methods of evaluation that the clinical team may employ. These tests include physical examinations and observations of movements of the mouth and throat or evaluations that include specialized equipment for imaging and recording the movements involved in voice, speech, and swallowing. These examinations are considered complementary and are often used in combination during the care of patients with head and neck cancer. Tests are selected by the speech-language pathologist and physician based on the condition of the patient, clinical setting, and questions that need to be answered regarding the patient's communication and swallowing function. It should be emphasized that all of these assessment procedures require specialized training by highly skilled and competent clinicians.

Non-instrumented Evaluation

The patient and caregivers are interviewed by the speech-language pathologist as part of the initial clinical examination to gain an understanding of their perspective on communication and swallowing ability. Voice, speech, and swallowing are often evaluated in the context of examination of the function of the structures of the face, mouth, and throat and during the patient's production of sounds, words, and sentences. Swallowing observations may be made as different consistencies of liquid and textures of food are presented. The speech-language pathologist gains an impression of the patient's potential need for speech and swallowing rehabilitation throughout the evaluation. Clinicians are not able to precisely predict the specific nature of a patient's function posttreatment; however, they are able to gain a good impression of the treatment outcome based on their rehabilitative experience with other patients undergoing similar types of treatment. The speech-language pathologist is also looking for clinical signs and symptoms that may indicate a need for further instrumented speech, voice, and swallowing evaluations (Logemann, 1998).

Instrumented Examinations

The primary instrumented examinations that patients will experience involve either a viewing, fiber-optic scope placed into the nose or mouth and passed to the upper throat or motion radiographic imaging of the motions of swallowing. The speech-language pathologist and physician often perform both of these evaluations but for different purposes. Surgeons use the examinations to assist them in diagnosing tumors and to survey structures during the posttreatment period. The speech-language pathologist, on the other hand, employs these viewing tools to gain an assessment of the functional outcome of the treatment, determine whether and how the patient can eat and drink safely, provide visual feedback to the patient during therapy, and monitor changes in function over time. The speech-language pathologist and otolaryngologist function as a team with the patient's recovery as their common goal regardless of the type of cancer treatment (Langmore, 2001; Logemann, 1998).

Communication and Swallowing Treatment

Appropriate and comprehensive speech and swallowing assessments should serve to drive the patient's treatment plan. No one treatment or management plan is appropriate for all patients. The selection of treatment should be based on scientific evidence that supports its impact on improving function and the nature and type of communication and swallowing problem observed during the evaluation. Other factors that play into the selection of appropriate treatments include nutrition, quality of life, the social and environmental circumstances of the patient, the degree of patient independence, and the goals of the patient and family.

Speech and voice intervention involves educating patients on the roles of the speech subsystems and teaching compensatory strategies or engaging the patient in active speech, voice, and swallowing exercises that maximize oral communication and swallowing ability. Instructions to optimize oral and vocal hygiene are often included as front-line methods to improve the overall comfort and effort associated with speech, voice, and swallowing. The patient may be taught methods to maximize the range, coordination, and speed of movement of oral-facial, pharyngeal, and laryngeal muscles. Further, they may be instructed in therapy techniques that enhance speech resonance and improve the quality and clarity of voice production. Patients are often instructed to initially slow their rate of speech and "overarticulate" to improve listener intelligibility. Some patients may benefit from oral prosthetics to replace resected structures or improve tongue-to-palate contact. Patients with extensive laryngeal cancer may require training with an alternative communication device such as an electrolarynx or voice prosthetics. Many patients may require temporary use of nonverbal methods of communication during the initial healing process, such as writing or picture boards, immediately following their surgery. A few patients may need long-term use of augmentative devices (Casper & Colton, 1998; Logemann, 1998; Lazarus, 2000; Stemple et al., 2000; Sullivan & Guilford, 1999; Ward & van As-Brooks, 2007).

Intervention for swallowing deficits often includes initial modification of liquid and food consistency, texture, and volume because studies and experience have demonstrated that the swallowing mechanism can be positively influenced by these alterations. The swallowing therapy program often integrates the effective use of postural modifications to the head, neck, and trunk during swallowing to take advantage of the alterations that gravity provides with these postures. Patients are often instructed in the use of special maneuvers to facilitate bolus flow, bolus clearance, and airway protection. Active exercises of muscles of the tongue and throat have also been shown to effectively impact the swallowing process in many patients. Techniques that facilitate heightened sensation in the mouth and throat may also be applied. Some patients will also benefit from adaptive feeding devices and oral appliances to assist them in placement and transport of liquid or food into and through the mouth (Lazarus, 2000; Logemann, 1998; Martin-Harris, 1999; Sullivan & Guilford, 1999; Ward & van As-Brooks, 2007).

In summary, multiple factors influence the degree of communication and swallowing difficulty that a patient will experience. The location and extent of disease, the method of treatment to address the disease, coexisting health issues, and motivation of the patient all affect functional outcome. Pretreatment evaluation and counseling is vital to preparing patients and their significant others for the challenges that result from head and neck cancer treatments. Appropriate and timely evaluations and early intervention are also critical factors directed toward optimizing the functional recovery of patients. Optimal recovery and maintenance of speech, voice, and swallowing function may require a lifetime effort of consciously engaging in exercises and compensation. These challenges are met through patient motivation, social support, specialized multidisciplinary team management, and continued advances in the science of rehabilitative methods.

References

Casper, J. K., & Colton, R. H. (1998). *Clinical manual for laryngectomy and head/neck rehabilitation* (2nd ed.). San Diego, CA: Singular.

Dikeman, K. J., & Kazandjian, M. S. (2003). *Communication and swallowing management of tracheostomized and ventilator dependent patients* (2nd ed.). Clifton Park, NY: Thompson Delmar Learning.

Langmore, S. (2001). *Endoscopic evaluation and treatment of swallowing disorders.* New York: Thieme.

Lazarus, C. L. (2000). Management of swallowing disorders in head and neck cancer patients: Optimal patterns of care. *Seminars in Speech and Language, 21*, 293–309.

Logemann, J.A. (1998). *Evaluation and treatment of swallowing disorders.* Austin: ProEd.

Logemann, J.A., Pauloski, B. R., Rademaker, A. W., Colangelo, L. A. (1997). Speech and swallowing rehabilitation for head and neck cancer patients. *Oncology (Williston Park), 11*(5), 651–656, 659; discussion 659, 663–654.

Martin-Harris, B. (1999). Treatment of dysphagia in adults: Methods and effects [Self-study videocassette program sponsored by the American Speech-Language Hearing Association]. Produced by Rehab Training Network—Broadcast September 16, 1999.

Mittal, B. B., Pauloski, B. R., Haraf, D. J., Pelzer, H. J., Argiris, A., Vokes, E. E., et al. (2003). Swallowing dysfunction—Preventative and rehabilitation strategies in patients with head-and-neck cancers treated with surgery, radiotherapy, and chemotherapy: A critical review. *International Journal of Radiation, Oncology, Biology, Physics, 57*, 1219–1230.

Pauloski, B. R., Rademaker, A. W., Logemann, J. A, & Colangelo, L. A. (1998). Speech and swallowing in irradiated and nonirradiated postsurgical oral cancer patients. *Otolaryngology—Head and Neck Surgery, 118*(5), 616–624.

Stemple, J. C., Glaze, L., & Gerderman, B. (2000). *Clinical voice pathology: Theory and management* (2nd ed.). San Diego, CA: Singular.

Sullivan, P. A., & Guilford, A. M. (1999). *Swallowing Intervention in Oncology*. San Diego, CA: Singular.

Ward, E. C., & van As-Brooks, C. J. (2007). *Head and neck cancer: Treatment, rehabilitation, and outcomes*. San Diego, CA: Plural.

Resources

Locating a Speech-Language Pathologist

The American Speech-Language-Hearing Association (ASHA). (Available at: http://www.asha.org)

Specialty Board on Swallowing and Swallowing Disorders (BRS-S). (Available at: http://www.swallowingdisorders.org)

Cookbooks

Achilles, E. (2004). *The dysphagia cookbook: Great tasting and nutritious recipes for people with swallowing difficulties*. Nashville, TN: Cumberland House. A specialty cookbook filled with nutritious, great-tasting recipes. (Available at: http://www.dysphagia.com)

Clegg, H., & Miletello, G. (2001). *Eating well through cancer: Easy recipes & recommendations during & after treatment*. Memphis, TN: Wimmer Cookbooks. Collection of 200 easy recipes to help cancer patients tolerate treatment. (Available at: http://www.amazon.com)

Dethero, B. R. (1999). *Let's do lunch*. Cleveland, TN: Dethero Enterprises. A handbook with nonchew recipes. (Available at: http://www.dinner throughastraw.net)

Katz, R. (2004). *One bite at a time: Nourishing recipes for cancer survivors and their friends*. Berkeley, CA: Celestial Arts. (Available at: http://www.amazon.com)

SPOHNC. (2005). *Eat well—stay nourished: A recipe and resource guide for coping with eating challenges*. Lenexa, KS: Cookbook Publishers. (Available at: http://www.spohnc.org)

Thigpen, P. A. (1999). *Dinner through a straw*. Cleveland, TN: Dethero Enterprises. A favorite handbook for patients of oral surgery and others who cannot chew. (Available at: http://www.dinnerthroughastraw.net)

Weihofen, D. L., & Marino, C. (1998). *The cancer survival cookbook: 200 quick ways with helpful eating hints.* Nourishing recipes and practical advice are provided to help cancer patients in their recovery. New York: John Wiley and Sons. (Available at: http://www.amazon.com)

Weihofen, D. L., & Robbins, J. (2002). *Easy-to-swallow, easy-to-chew cookbook.* New York: John Wiley and Sons. Packed with more than 150 tasty and nutritious recipes for people who have difficulty swallowing. (Available at: http://www.amazon.com)

Wilson, J. R. (2003). *The I can't chew cookbook.* Alameda, CA: Hunter House. (Available at: http://www.amazon.com)

Womack, P. (1999). Everything you need to know to cope with your own or a loved one's dysphagia. *The dysphagia challenge.* (Available at: http://www.dysphagiabooks.com)

Wright, C. (2005). *Second helpings.* Salem, VA: Author. Recipes (75) developed by caregiver for her husband who has difficulty chewing and swallowing. (Available at: http://www.secondhelpingsbycacky.com)

Resources for Thickening Agents

Med-Diet: http://www.dysphagia-diet.com

Novartis: Resource® Thickenup:
http://www.dysphagia-diet.com/novartis.htm

Hormel HealthLabs:
http://www.dysphagia-diet.com/hhl.htm

Hydra~Aid Gel Liquid Thickener:
http://www.thickitretail.com

Diafoods: Thick-It®
Milani Foods, 800-333-0003
East of the Mississippi: Health Call at 800-778-5704
West of the Mississippi: Kansas Specialty Service at
877-751-5095
http://www.thickitdelivered.com
http://www.walgreens.com
http://www.brucemedical.com/thickit.htm
Thickens hot, cold, and pureed foods. Pharmacies will
order for you.

Regular Instant Thickener
Nutra/Balance Company
155 Wadsworth Way
Indianapolis, IN 46219
800-654-3691 or 317-356-5478
http://www.nutra-balance-products.com

Resources for Modified Feeding Utensils and Cups

RehabMart, LLC
150 Sagewood Drive
Winterville, GA 30683-1563
800-827-8283 (toll free)
706-213-1144 (direct)
603-843-2144 (fax)
http://www.rehabmart.com/category/Dining_Aids.htm

Zip-N-Squeeze
Susan Beaudette, RN
P.O. Box 575
Yerba Linda, CA 92885
714-997-7146
http://www.zip-n-squeeze.com

8

MEETING THE CHALLENGES OF GOOD NUTRITION

Jennifer Thompson, RD, LD, CNSD

This chapter on nutrition aims to provide useful information to patients with oral and head and neck cancer and their caregivers. While this information may be well known to some, it may be the first time others have considered what they eat as more than something to satisfy cravings. After reading this chapter, you should be able to understand why nutrition is important and how it can be included in the fight against cancer.

Good Nutrition for Oral and Head and Neck Cancer Patients

The definition of "good" nutrition varies depending on an individual's circumstances. The ideal or most beneficial dietary intake for the public is not always the best diet for those who have cancer. During cancer treatment the nutritional needs of a person are usually higher than normal. This means if someone required 2,000 calories a day before being diagnosed with cancer, the need may increase to 2,500 or 3,000 calories a day during treatment. One way to measure whether you are eating adequately is to follow your weight on a weekly basis. If your weight stays the same or is stable, then you are probably eating well enough (unless you are retaining fluid). If you start to see weight loss, then it may be time to make some changes.

Even if individuals are overweight, it is still important for them to consume adequate calories. Many people think, "I have extra weight to lose. I'll be OK." However, cancer alters the body's metabolism as do stressful situations such as undergoing chemotherapy and/or radiation. Thus, muscle wasting occurs along with fat loss, leaving patients weak at a time when they need strength.

A Balanced Diet

Table 8–1 details what a balanced diet looks like. Basically, it means eating a variety of foods every day. Nutrients are found in many different foods, yet each food group also contains nutrients that are unique to that group. In addition, one group may be a better source of nutrients than another group. For example, iron found in leafy

Table 8–1. USDA Guidelines* for 2,000 Calories per Day Diet

Food Group	Servings Per Day
Fruit	2 cups
Vegetables	2½ cups
Grains	6 ounces
Meats/beans	5½ ounces
Milk	3 cups
Oil	6 teaspoons
"Discretionary" or free to choose	270 calories

*Released in 2005 after thorough review of latest scientific research.

Go to http://www.mypyramid.gov to find out your personal needs.

green vegetables is poorly absorbed, but iron found in red meat is an excellent source because it is absorbed very well. Therefore, any diet that requires you to eliminate a food group completely should be carefully examined. Talk to your health care provider if you are considering following a new diet or if you are having difficulty with your current diet. Your ability to eat a balanced diet in the amounts recommended may be limited, and the means by which nutrition is obtained may need to be altered. A registered dietitian (RD) is an expert in all aspects of nutrition. If your cancer center does not have an RD on staff, go to http:www.eatright.org to locate one in your area.

Why Nutrition Is Important

There is evidence that maintaining a well-nourished body helps a person handle a treatment regimen better. "Research shows that poor nutritional status and inadequate dietary intake have a negative impact on outcomes of cancer therapy, including increased risk for complications, poor tolerance, and response to treatment and a lower quality of life" (Jacobsen, 2006).

Screening Head and Neck Patients for Nutritional Risk

The following signs or symptoms place a cancer patient at risk for malnutrition:

- Weight loss (unintentional)
- Loss of appetite (referred to as anorexia in medical terms)
- Difficulty chewing or swallowing (referred to as dysphagia)
- Poor dietary intake (usually related to loss of appetite and difficulty chewing or swallowing)
- Feeling full quickly when eating
- Nausea, vomiting, or diarrhea that persists for more than a day or two
- Oral mucositis secondary to radiation therapy and chemotherapy

Nutritional Therapy

Nutritional therapy involves using the diet to achieve a certain goal. During cancer treatment, the main goal of nutrition is to support patients so they are able to withstand the surgery, radiation, and/or chemotherapy. A poor diet can cause patients to have their cancer treatment stopped or postponed temporarily if they are too weak to handle treatment-related stress. It can also delay the healing process once the treatment is completed.

Maintaining Good Nutrition During Treatment

Attitude plays a key role in the ability to maintain good nutrition during treatment. When you are physically worn out and if you experience any of the symptoms listed previously, you may struggle with eating or drinking anything, much less everything your body needs. Your general mind-set will be important. If you believe nutrition is vital to your success during treatment, you will be more likely to make yourself do more than you thought possible. A pro-nutrition mind-set may have other benefits, such as causing less friction when caregivers are encouraging you to eat or when health care providers are giving recommendations for using a feeding tube.

The Role of Vitamins and Minerals

Vitamins, minerals, and phytonutrients play a variety of roles in the daily functions of the body and are as necessary as carbohydrates, protein, and fat. Without adequate vitamins and minerals, the body is unable to fully utilize the calories consumed. However, high intakes of vitamins and minerals can be unsafe during active treatment and are not generally recommended. Before you start your treatment, talk with your health care provider about any vitamin or mineral supplements you are already taking or considering. Some cancer centers will advise *not* to take any supplements, even a general multivitamin, during days of radiation or chemotherapy. Outside of radiation and chemotherapy days, a general multivitamin with minerals that contains no more than 100% RDA (recommended dietary allowance) should be sufficient.

Herbal Supplements

Talk with your health care provider *before* you start taking any herbal supplements. Many herbal supplements have interactions with medicines, including chemotherapy drugs, which may be undesirable. Additionally, herbs from foreign countries are not regulated. If your doctor is unfamiliar with the supplements you are interested in taking, the dietitian or pharmacist may be able to provide information for you on their safety during treatment. Any information you read about dietary or herbal supplements must be carefully examined. Go to http://www.quackwatch.com or http://www.mskcc.org/about herbs for information about these supplements.

Feeding Tubes

Your doctor may suggest that a feeding tube be put in place before you begin treatment to provide a route for water, nutrition, and medicines when you are unable to adequately consume these substances orally. A feeding tube is a necessary tool because the mouth and/or throat may become very sore during cancer treatment involving surgery, radiation, and/or chemotherapy. The length of treatment may vary, as may the time for healing, from several weeks to several months. Thus, the feeding tube provides a way for you to give your body the nourishment it needs to withstand the treatment and to recover as quickly as possible. You may use the feeding tube occasionally in the beginning, but it may eventually become the only way you are able to get water and "food." If you are still wary about its value, consider it a potential stress-reliever. With a feeding tube, you and your caregivers won't have to worry about how you are going to drink or eat when there is discomfort in your mouth and throat. There is adequate evidence in the medical literature to show that patients who are malnourished do not respond as well to chemotherapy or radiation therapy.

Supplementing the Diet to Maintain Balance

When food no longer appeals to you or when it is too painful to chew and swallow, then it is time to consider nutritional supplements. If you find yourself struggling with eating from a lack of appetite, then supplements come in handy because drinking may be an easier and quicker way to get in the calories. If you start to develop sores in the mouth and throat but are still able to tolerate liquids, then supplements can provide a concentrated source of nutrition. If you find yourself unable to tolerate anything by mouth, supplements may be put into the feeding tube.

Supplements are divided into those intended to be consumed by mouth and those that are meant to be given through a feeding tube.

Oral Supplements

These supplements can be given through the feeding tube as well. Most supplements contain a combination of fat, protein, carbohydrates, vitamins, and minerals. However, there are supplements that contain only protein to help patients who are unable to meet the demands for protein because they are unable to tolerate chicken, beef, pork, fish, and seafood. The remaining discussion will focus on those supplements that contain a combination of nutrients. See Table 8–2 at the end of the section for specific information on current supplements available.

Clear liquid or "milky." Many people are surprised to learn that there are clear liquid supplements available. They are often described as juicelike with the added benefit of having protein added to them. The "milky" supplements are more common, but they are not all milk based. Some use soy milk instead of cow's milk. Regardless of the milk used, all supplements are lactose free.

Powder or ready to drink. There are versions that come in powder form and require some liquid to make them tolerable. The ready-to-drink versions are available in cans or resealable bottles. Unopened they can be kept at room temperature or refrigerated, but they should be kept in the refrigerator after opening.

Regular, plus, high protein. To add further to the decision-making process, you will find different names for the same basic product. The "regular" option is the base model and contains approximately 240 calories and 10 grams of protein. The "plus" option contains more calories and protein, approximately 350 calories and 13 to 15 grams of protein per serving. The "high protein" option usually keeps the calories about the same as the "regular" but adds more protein. There are even some supplements that contain 560 to 600 calories.

Brand name or generic. The common brand-name supplements that most people are familiar with are Ensure and Boost. Anybody who has tried either one will be glad to share their opinion, but try them for yourself and see which one you like best. Most people end up preferring one over the other. A few will like both and some dislike both. Fortunately, they are not the only supplements on the market. There are other products, including generic versions that are usually more economical.

Tube Feed Supplements

One big difference between these supplements and the oral alternatives is the lack of flavor. Otherwise, these supplements are the same in content. The choices to be made among these formulas include calorie content and any special ingredients or formulations. For calories, the range is typically from 240 to 480 per can. This affects you in two ways: (a) the number of cans needed to meet your needs and (b) the amount of water provided to help with hydration. Two examples of special ingredients are fiber and omega-3 fatty acids. Some supplements contain formulas that are disease specific such as those designed for patients with renal or kidney disease.

Your dietitian can assist you in determining the best formula for you and your unique situation and may be able to provide you with samples of supplements. You can try different brands and flavors to see which ones suit you or which ones work best as a tube feeding.

Throughout this section the who, what, when, where, and why of nutrition have been discussed so that patients and caregivers may be better equipped for their fight against cancer. A well-nourished body will be able to better withstand the surgery, radiation, and/or chemotherapy treatment. Here is a good visual comparison to help you remember the importance of nutrition: Imagine yourself as a car. No one expects a car to run on empty. It must be filled with gas on a regular basis to run effectively. Food is your fuel to keep you running well.

The information provided in this section is not all-inclusive. Your local dietitian will be glad to work with you on a one-on-one basis to personalize your nutrition. You should not be hesitant to ask your doctor for a referral to a dietitian. If the facility where you are receiving treatment does not have a dietitian available, you can find one on http://www.eatright.org.

Table 8–2. Nutritional Supplements

Novartis Products

Novartis products are available at stores unless indicated by *; online sites include http://www.boost.com and http://www.walgreens.com; phone numbers are 800-828-9194 (Walgreens), 800-438-6153 (TAD), and 800-446-6380 (Redline).

Product	Flavors	Cal	Prot	Fiber	Admin
Benecalorie	Unflavored	330	7 g	0	Oral
Boost	Multi	240	10 g	0	Oral
Boost Plus	Multi	360	14 g	0	Oral
Boost High Protein	Multi	240	15 g	0	Oral
Boost Glucose Control (DM)	Multi	190	16 g	3 g	Oral
Boost Pudding (DM)	Van, choc, butterscotch	240	7 g	0	Oral
Boost Hi-Protein Powder*	Van	200	13 g	0	Oral
Nutrament* (12 oz)	Multi	360	16 g	0	Oral
Resource Support*	Multi	360	21 g	3 g	Oral
Resource 2.0*	Van, orange crème	475	21 g	0	Oral
Resource Shake*	Van	270	9 g	0	Oral
Resource Shake plus*	Multi	480	15 g	0	Oral
Resource Fruit Flavored beverage*	Multi	250	9 g	0	Oral
Ultracal*	Unflavored	250	10.7 g	3.4 g	Tube

Table 8–2. *continued*

Nestle Products

Nestle products are generally ordered online or by phone; the CIB powder is available in stores as well. Online sites include http://www.carnationinstantbreakfast.com and http://www.nestle-nutrition.com.

Product	Flavors	Cal	Prot	Fiber	Admin
Carnation Instant Breakfast (CIB) powder	St, choc, van	130	5 g	0	Oral
CIB Plus	St, choc, van	375	13 g	0	Oral
CIB Very High Calorie (VHC)	Van only	560	23 g	0	Oral
CIB juice drink	Sweet berry, orange	163	6.5 g	0	Oral
Nutren Probalance	Van	300	13.5 g	2.5 g	Oral/tube
Nutren Replete	Van	250	15.6 g	3.4 g	Oral/tube

There are a variety of Nutren products that vary in calorie level, fiber content, and indications for use. Your dietitian can help you determine which one is right for you.

Ross Products

Ross products are available at stores unless indicated by *; online sites include http://www.ross.com. Phone number: 800-986-8502.

Product	Flavors	Cal	Prot	Fiber	Admin
Ensure	Multi	250	9 g	0	Oral
Ensure Plus	Multi	350	13 g	0	Oral
Ensure High Protein	Multi	230	12 g	0	Oral
Ensure Fiber	Van, choc	250	8.8 g	2.8 g	Oral
Ensure Pudding (8 oz)	Multi	340	8 g	2 g	Oral
Glucerna Shake (DM)	Multi	220	10 g	2.8 g	Oral

continues

Table 8–2. *continued*

Ross Products *continued*

Product	Flavors	Cal	Prot	Fiber	Admin
Juven*	Grape, orange	78	14 g	0	Oral
Jevity* (also comes in variations with more calories and protein for the same volume)	Unflavored	250	10.4 g	3.4 g	Oral/tube
Osmolite* (also comes in variations with more calories and protein for the same volume)	Unflavored	250	8.8 g	0	Oral/tube
Two Cal HN*	Van, butter pecan	475	20 g	1.2 g	Oral/tube

OTHER SUPPLEMENTS

Scandipharm (Axcan pharma)
Phone 800-472-2634; http://www.scandishake.com

Product	Flavors	Cal	Prot	Fiber	Admin
Scandishake	Multi	600	6 g	0	Oral
Scandical (tablespoon)	Unflavored	35	0	0	Oral

Nutra/Balance
Phone 800-654-3691; http://www.nutra-balance-products.com

Product	Flavors	Cal	Prot	Fiber	Admin
Nutra/Balance 2.0	Multi	470	20 g	0	Oral
Nutra/Shake Supreme	Multi	400	12 g	0	Oral
Nutra/Shake Fruit Plus	Multi	400	12 g	0	Oral

Table 8–2. *continued*

Resurgex
Phone 877-737-8749; www.resurgex.com

Product	Flavors	Cal	Prot	Fiber	Admin
Resurgex	Van, fruit blast	90	12 g	0	Oral
Resurgex Plus	Van, choc	400	21 g	0	Oral
Resurgex Select	Multi	350	15 g	0	Oral

Protein Powder Options

Product	Flavors	Cal	Prot	Fiber	Admin
Resource Beneprotein (Novartis) 1 scoop	Unflavored	25	6 g	0	Oral
EvoPro 1 scoop (http://www.cytosport.com)	Multi	140	26 g	0	Oral
Mega-Isolate 2 scoops (GNC) http://www.gnc.com	Van, choc	230	50 g	1 g	Oral

Weight Gainer Powder Options

Product	Flavors	Cal	Prot	Fiber	Admin
Weight Gainer 1850 (GNC) http://www.gnc.com 3 cups powder mixed with 3 cups 2% milk	Multi	1,850	74 g	0	Oral

continues

Table 8–2. *continued*

Weight Gainer Powder Options *continued*

Product	Flavors	Cal	Prot	Fiber	Admin
Russian Bear 5000 (suggested to mix with 1 gallon of whole milk to reach 5,000 calories) http://www.nicemuscle.com	Van, choc	2,600	184 g	0	Oral
Twinlab Mass Fuel (suggested to mix 4 scoops to 3 cups milk) http://www.nicemuscle.com	Van, choc	600	50 g	0	Oral

Products with (DM) are lower in total carbohydrates and specifically made for people with diabetes. However, many of the other supplements can still be used by people with diabetes. A dietitian can help you determine the best fit for you. Often the timing and amount of supplement consumed at each time can be modified to allow most of these products to be used.

Product nutrient values and ingredients are subject to change. See the product label or contact the manufacturer for the most current information. This information was updated May 2007.

To locate a dietitian or nutritionist, you may request a referral from your physician or contact the American Dietetic Association (http://www.eatright.org).

DISCLAIMER: This product data is provided to readers as a convenience and guide only. **SPOHNC does not recommend nor endorse** any product listed herein. Consult your physician prior to using any of the products aforementioned.

Reference

Jacobsen, M. (2006, Spring). Getting the word out: Nutrition counseling improves outcomes. *Oncology Nutrition Connection, 14*(2).

9

MEETING THE CHALLENGES OF INSURANCE ISSUES

A. HEALTH INSURANCE IN THE UNITED STATES

Beth Darnley, CPO, Connie Slayton, BSN
Constance Goodman, RN,
Tanya Walker, RN, BSN
Mary Giguere, RN, BSN, Tami Lewis, RN

Advances in medical technology and medicine make health insurance a necessity in the 21st century. People are living longer, the aging population is rising, and unfortunately data shows that as we become more technically advanced we are also moving away from healthier lifestyles.

Most Americans obtain health insurance coverage through an employer as part of a group health benefit. Employer-sponsored group health plans must cover all employees regardless of their medical history. There is an open enrollment period, decided by the employer, at which time all employees who have not yet signed up for insurance have the ability to do so. The insurance carrier can impose a preexisting condition clause on individuals who do not have credible coverage (an example would be a person who has a 63-day or greater lapse in coverage). This clause is typically 12 months in duration and at 12 months and 1 day the person is covered the same as any other insured employee. The clause will exclude charges for the preexisting condition(s) only. Most employer-sponsored group health plans are federally regulated by the Employee Retirement Income Security Act of 1974 (ERISA). ERISA outlines the appellant process for appealing a claim. Another benefit of employer-sponsored group health plans is that insured employees can elect to continue their group coverage if they leave their employer. Federal law mandates that employers with 20 or more employees must offer COBRA, the Consolidated Omnibus Budget Reconciliation Act. Additional information on both programs will be reviewed at the end of this chapter.

If you are self-employed, check to see whether your state has any health insurance companies that offer group health plans for groups of one. This will vary by state, and requirements will vary by insurance company. To learn whether your state offers this coverage, contact a local insurance agent and/or the National Association for the Self-Employed (http://www.nase.org).

You may be able to purchase an individual insurance plan depending on your medical history. If you have had a previous health condition, you may face a preexisting condition waiting period. The length of the waiting period must be disclosed to you if it is imposed. Individual plans are subject to state laws. Another alternative is to see whether your state offers risk pool coverage, which provides health insurance options for high-risk individuals. These are state programs that serve people with preexisting health conditions who are often denied or find it difficult to obtain affordable coverage in the private market. To learn more about what your state offers, contact your state insurance commissioner at http://www.insure.com, who can provide information specific to your state.

When you sign up for health insurance—just like when you sign your auto or homeowner's policies—you are entering into a contract with the insurance carrier. Regardless of who your insurance carrier is or what type of insurance you have, you are subject to the terms of your policy. It is very important that you read your plan carefully. If you have questions about any portion of your policy, refer to the phone number provided on your insurance card.

Many patients are surprised to find themselves facing large out-of-pocket expenses even though they are "fully insured." Usual, customary, and reasonable (UCR) charges are often one reason for this situation. UCR rates are established based on the geographic region in which you live and the specific service provided to you.

Network Providers and UCRs

Most health insurance policies covering Americans today use a specified "network" of providers. Whether you have a health maintenance organization (HMO), a preferred provider organization (PPO), a point of service (POS) plan, or another variant of one of these plans, you generally have the most extensive coverage when you visit a physician or medical facility that participates in your insurance carrier's network. These providers may include physicians, hospitals, outpatient diagnostic facilities, radiation therapy centers, outpatient infusion centers, or any other provider of medical services. When you remain within your provider network, you are not responsible for UCR rates and charges. Your insurance carrier is responsible for annually providing beneficiaries with a listing of participating providers.

When your insurance carrier receives a claim on your behalf, it processes claims payments per the terms of the contract. Once the claim has been processed, the provider and the patient both receive statements more commonly referred to as an "explanation of benefits" (EOB). It is important to review each EOB you receive because EOBs will tell you the amounts paid to the provider as well as any financial responsibility you may have.

Out-of-Network Providers and UCRs

Patients often make the choice to go to providers not participating in their network. If you choose to do this, it is critical to make sure that you have out-of-network (OON) benefits under your policy. If you do not have OON benefits and you elect to receive care at an OON facility, you may not receive *any* insurance reimbursement. If you have OON benefits, your claim will be processed using the prevailing UCR rates for the services provided. In addition, the provider may "balance bill" you for the difference between what the physician charges and what the insurance company pays.

As the following example illustrates, the amount of patient financial responsibility can be much greater than originally anticipated. The application of UCR rates and balance billing can more than double the patient's financial responsibility.

Example:

OON facility bills actual charge	$1,000
UCR allowable charge	$400
60% (OON) insurance paid	$240
Your 40% coinsurance	$160
Balance billing choosing OON	$600
Your total costs	$760

Even if your policy has an out-of-pocket maximum, it is important to understand that *only* your portion of the UCR amount allowed is applied toward your maximum. In the example just given, only $160 (your portion of the amount the insurance company deemed payable) of the $760 you paid is counted toward your yearly out-of-pocket maximum. For this reason many patients have much larger than anticipated medical bills when seeking services at an OON provider.

Medicare and UCRs

UCR charges are not regulated by state or federal agencies, but Medicare does publish its UCR fee schedule. This is commonly referred to as Medicare allowable charges. Providers who participate with Medicare agree to accept the Medicare allowable charge as full payment. Bear in mind that the patient will be responsible for the coinsurance and deductible.

Example:

Chemotherapy actual charge	$500
UCR allowable charge	$300
Medicare 80/20 insurance paid	$240
Your 20% coinsurance	$60
Your total costs	$60

Medicare providers may choose not to bill the patient for amounts above the Medicare allowable fee schedule. It is important to verify that your provider "accepts Medicare assignment" or is a "Medicare provider" to avoid unexpected and potentially large out-of-pocket expenses.

Sometimes, a health care provider will notify patients—either verbally or by written notification—that they may be subject to balance billing after the insurance carrier has paid the allowable charge or if the claim is denied completely for reimbursement. This communication constitutes a "waiver of financial responsibility." This happens most commonly when a health care provider anticipates that the insurance carrier may deny a claim and the physician and patient want to proceed with the therapy regardless of the insurance coverage.

All insurers, including Medicare, provide an appeals process for denial of service. To understand more about these processes, please refer to *Your Guide to the Appeals Process* from the Patient Advocate Foundation (PAF) or contact PAF directly at 800-532-5274.

Employee Retirement Income Security Act of 1974 (ERISA)

ERISA is a federal law that was established to protect the rights of employees and the security of their retirement funds and medical benefits provided by an employer. ERISA sets minimum standards for most voluntarily established pension and health plans in private industry to provide protection for individuals in these plans.

In general, ERISA covers any employer with a retirement plan and/or employee benefit plan. Only a few plans are exempt, such as group health plans established or maintained by governmental entities (federal, state, and local government); church plans; or plans that are maintained solely to comply with applicable workers' compensation, unemployment, or disability laws. ERISA also does not cover plans maintained outside the United States primarily for the benefit of nonresident aliens or unfunded excess benefit plans. For more information about ERISA, visit http://www.dol.gov/dol/topic/health-plans/index.htm

Amendments to ERISA

There have been a number of amendments to ERISA, expanding the protections available to health benefit plan participants and beneficiaries. One important amendment, the Consolidated Omnibus Budget Reconciliation Act (COBRA), provides some workers and their families with the right to continue their health coverage for a period of 18 months, with an extension option of an additional 11 months in certain circumstances, after specified events, such as the loss of a job. Another amendment to ERISA is the Health Insurance Portability and Accountability Act (HIPAA), which provides important new protections for working Americans and their families and who have group benefits and who might otherwise be uninsurable. Other important amendments include the Newborns' and Mothers' Health Protection Act, the Mental Health Parity Act, and the Women's Health and Cancer Rights Act.

Requirements of Employers

ERISA requires that sponsors of private employee benefit plans provide participants and beneficiaries with adequate information regarding their plans. In addition, under the ERISA law, your employer must provide you with a copy of your summary plan description (SPD) and plan documents within 120 days after the plan becomes effective. The plan administrator must also distribute SPDs to participants and beneficiaries every 5 years unless no changes have occurred, at which time the administrator may wait 10 years. If a beneficiary requests a copy of the SPD and/or complete plan language in writing, it must be supplied within 30 days after receiving the written request. The request must be made to the plan administrator with reference to the ERISA law. Failure to comply can result in a penalty of up to $100 per day and is governed by the Department of Labor.

Under ERISA an employer is required to provide adequate notice to a plan participant whose claim for benefits has been denied. In the case of group health or disability plans, the notice must contain information about any internal rules, guidelines, or protocols that were relied upon when making the decision. The denial letter must outline "the specific reason for such denial, written in a manner calculated to be understood by the plan participant." For example, if the decision is based on a plan limitation that excludes treatments that are not medically necessary or are experimental, the notice must explain that scientific or clinical reason for the decision. In addition, the plan participant must be given "a reasonable opportunity . . . for a full and fair review (ERISA Sec. 1133)." Under ERISA regulations, a denial of any claim for benefits must be made "within a reasonable period of time." As a general rule, a period of more than 90 days is deemed unreasonable. If circumstances require a longer processing time, the plan may request an extension up to an additional 90 days after the participant has been given notice. When an urgent case is in need of an expedited decision, the plan must make its determination "as soon as possible, taking into account the medial exigencies" but no later than 72 hours after receipt of the claim unless the claim does not provide enough information to make a determination. The Department of Labor emphasizes that no time extensions are allowed in urgent cases. The determination of whether a claim is considered urgent can be made by a person acting on behalf of the plan "applying the judgment of a prudent layperson possesses an average knowledge of health and medicine." In addition, the plan must notify the patient within 45 days if a benefit claim is incomplete and specify the information required to complete the claim. The participant must be given at least 180 days to complete the claim. It is important that both the plan and the patient follow the deadlines given for appeal. In many cases the plan will no longer view the case if the deadline has passed.

Contact ERISA

ERISA plans are enforced by the Department of Labor's Employee Benefits Security Administration (EBSA). You may contact your local office by calling 866-444-3272 or review plans at http://www. dol.gov/dol/topic/health-plans/index.htm It is important to note that under ERISA, if consumers are denied treatment, they may be able to collect punitive damages or compensation only if their state has mandated that right under state law. For more information concerning your state's legal healthcare provisions, visit http://info. insure.com/health/lawtool.cfm.

Health Insurance Portability and Accountability Act (HIPAA)

HIPAA provides protections for beneficiaries covered by group health plans. It limits exclusions for preexisting conditions. It prohibits discrimination against employees and dependents based on their health status, and it guarantees renewability and availability of health coverage to certain employees and individuals. To be protected under HIPAA, there cannot be a lapse or break in coverage of more than 62 days.

Once members are no longer covered by a plan, they will be issued a certificate of credible coverage to provide to the new carrier. To learn more about your protections under HIPAA, visit http://www.dol.gov/dol/topic/health-plans/index.htm.

Consolidated Omnibus Budget Reconciliation Act (COBRA)

Certain employers with 20 or more full-time employees or equivalent in the previous 12 months are required to offer continuation of coverage under COBRA to qualified beneficiaries. A qualified beneficiary is any individual covered by the plan the day before the qualifying event. There are five qualifying events for which COBRA election would be necessary:

■ Voluntary or involuntary termination of employment for reasons other than "gross misconduct"
■ Reduction in the number of hours of employment
■ Divorce or legal separation of the covered employee
■ Death of the covered employee
■ Loss of "dependent child" status under the plan rules

Each beneficiary can elect COBRA independently. To learn more about your rights under COBRA, visit http://www.dol. gov/dol/topic/health-plans/index.htm.

Maintaining credible coverage is a concern for any individual, but to a patient diagnosed with a progressive disease, it is critical. Under HIPAA, beneficiaries covered by group health plans are safeguarded. A student will have to be diligent in maintaining group health coverage. Under private or individual plans, the insurer may impose a complete preexisting exclusion of anything related to your critical diagnosis. For patients facing coverage concerns, seek the assistance of a professional case manager at the Patient Advocate Foundation at 800-532-5274 or via the Internet at help@patient advocate.org.

Individuals who do not have health insurance coverage and are in need of diagnostic services should contact their local health department. Patients diagnosed through certain programs may be entitled to immediate coverage through state or federal reimbursement programs.

If you lose your group health coverage benefits, check with your local Medicaid office to determine whether your children are eligible for coverage through SCHIPS (Children's Health Insurance Program). This program is typically administered on a sliding fee scale, allowing parents to have a higher income. For more information visit http://www.insurekidsnow.gov.

Medicaid

Medicaid is a federally and state funded, state-run program that provides medical coverage for individuals and families with limited income and resources that meet certain eligibility guidelines. Medicaid coverage varies from state to state, so a person who is eligible for Medicaid in one state may not be eligible in another state and the services provided by one state may differ from those provided in another state. Check with your local social services agency to see whether you qualify. For many uninsured individuals, the cost of health insurance is prohibitive. Check with your local Medicaid office to find out whether your state offers a HIPP (Health Insurance Premium Payment) program.

Financial Assistance

If you have not yet started treatment, you may want to find a facility that offers charity care or has a financial assistance program. Call the billing office of a selected facility and ask whether they have a hardship, charity, or an indigent program. These are most likely found at public hospitals and faith-based facilities. Be prepared to offer the facility details about your health and financial status.

There are many programs available to assist you with getting your medications. Many medications are available through patient assistance programs offered by the pharmaceutical companies. Each company has its own eligibility requirements and applications. You can visit http://www.needymeds.com or http://www.helping patients.com for complete listings of all drugs available through indigent programs.

The many facets of health care insurance discussed in this chapter are of great importance to the people of the United States, especially to the millions of patients and caregivers who are faced with illnesses and subsequent access difficulties. In today's world, it is imperative that patients or caregivers be provided with information in order to make the right decisions that can ultimately affect the health, long-term insurability, and financial stability of the individual. The following resources are intended to help provide additional information on some of these facets of health care insurance.

Consumer Guides

The Georgetown University Health Policy Institute has written *A Consumer Guide to Getting and Keeping Health Insurance* for each state and Washington, DC. These guides summarize key consumer rights and protections in job-based group health insurance and individually purchased coverage. They also alert consumers to public programs in each state that may provide or subsidize health coverage. For more information visit www.healthinsuranceinfo.net.

Government Web Sites

State insurance: http://www.naic.org/state_web_map.htm

ERISA: http://www.dol.gov/dol/topic/health-plans/index.htm.

COBRA: http://www.dol.gov/dol/topic/health-plans/index.htm.

HIPAA: http://www.dol.gov/dol/topic/health-plans/index.htm.

Medicare and Medicaid: http://www.cms.hhs.gov

Cost-Sharing Assistance Charities

Chronic Disease Fund
877-968-7233
http://www.cdfund.org

HealthWell Foundation
800-675-8416
http://www.healthwellfoundation.org

National Organization for Rare Disorders
866-828-8902
http://www.rarediseases.org

Patient Access Network
866-316-7263
http://www.patientaccessnetwork.org

Patient Advocate Foundation
866-512-3861
http://www.patientadvocate.org

Patient Services Inc.
800-366-7741
http://www.uneedpsi.org

Patient Assistance Program

RxAssist Patient Assistance Program Center. RxAssist is a pharmaceutical access information center created by Volunteers in Health Care (VIH). It is a resource center with information about patient assistance programs, Medicare Part D, programs for low-cost medications, and any other issues related to pharmaceutical access. Phone: 401-729-3284. Web site: http://www.rxassist.org.

Partnership for Prescription Assistance brings together America's pharmaceutical companies, doctors, other health care providers, patient advocacy organizations, and community groups to help qualifying patients who lack prescription coverage get the medicines they need through the public or private program that's right for them. Phone: 800-477-2669. Web site: http://www.pparx.org.

NeedyMeds is a 501(3)(c) nonprofit organization that provides information about assistance programs that help with the cost of medicine and other health care expenses. The information at NeedyMeds is available anonymously and free of charge. Web site: http://www.needymeds.com.

Together Rx Access is a free prescription savings program for eligible individuals and families who lack prescription drug coverage, are not eligible for Medicare, and are legal residents of the United States or Puerto Rico. Phone: 800-444-4106. Web site: http://www.togetherrxaccess.com.

B. MEDICALLY NECESSARY DENTAL CARE

Mary Kaye Richter and Malinda Heuring

Adapted from information prepared by
the National Foundation for Ectodermal Dysplasias

"These charges are not covered under your medical plan. Please submit them to your dental carrier." How familiar these words are to the oral and head and neck cancer survivor who is undergoing rehabilitative treatment by an oral surgeon, dentist, or prosthodontist to restore functions of speech and mastication to an acceptable state.

The fact that the patient was diagnosed with oral and head and neck cancer and that the dental problems and rehabilitation program occurred as a result of necessary medical treatment for the cancer is often lost as insurance companies attempt to fit the patient into the "mold" that has been created. Granted, under normal circumstances dental services and supplies provided by the dental team are excluded from medical insurance plans; however, in cases in which dental care is necessitated by a treatment and/or surgery for a medical problem, there should be no question of medical insurance benefits.

Oral and head and neck cancer patients have a wide range of challenges they must address during their cancer journey. One of these challenges is dental care and proving that the care is medically necessary and therefore covered under a medical insurance policy. Proving that dental care is medically necessary is not easy. It is helpful to have a record of having received medical benefits for oral and head and neck cancer treatments prior to seeking dental benefits under the medical policy. Begin your quest with the very first visit to the dentist.

When dealing with your insurer, it is important to keep detailed records. Start a notebook that will allow you to document all telephone conservations with the insurance company. Request that all rulings be made in writing and file this documentation with your notebook. The process ahead may not be an easy one, but keeping duplicates of all letters and notes from all telephone conversations with the insurance company could ultimately prove helpful.

The first request for dental benefits from a medical insurance carrier is almost always denied. Typically, these requests are received by a clerk who is familiar with the policy language. Because dental benefits routinely excluded, the clerk will indicate that benefits do not apply and a denial will follow. You need this denial in writing.

Under the Employee Retirement and Income Security Act (ERISA), your denial letter should include a *specific reason* for the denial and a reference to your plan explaining the basis for the denial. After you receive this documentation, you can start the appeals process. When you appeal, you should immediately ask that a case manager handle your requests. A case manager is more capable of handling complex benefit questions.

Sometimes the process must be repeated . . . and repeated . . . and repeated. The average insurance clerk is not familiar with oral and head and neck cancer and serves the company not the consumer. It is important that the company understand that you will not give up until an appropriate decision is made. This can take many, many months. Customers are likely to either accept the initial denial or get tired of the fight. If success seems out of reach, the assistance of an attorney may be helpful. It doesn't take an insurer long to figure out that legal bills will quickly exceed the cost of a set of dentures and that it may be easier to pay the latter rather than the former. In addition, the situation could turn into a public relations nightmare for the company.

In either event, it is of the utmost importance that the insurance company be made to understand that oral and head and neck cancer and its treatments of radiation therapy and chemotherapy may result in dental problems and therefore the dental treatment for those problems should be considered a component of care necessitated by a medical condition.

If you receive insurance through an employer, be familiar with the type of insurance you have. Call the human resources manager or office manager and ask for that person's help in explaining your coverage. If the employer is self-insured, the employer typically hires a third party to administer the plan and the company pays the claims. This has its advantages and disadvantages.

If your company is self-insured, your company does not have to comply with the health insurance regulations in your state pursuant to ERISA. The employer can choose to pay a claim that typically is not a covered benefit. Work with the human resources department and explain your situation, both verbally and in writing. The company may choose to pay the claim, or the human resources department may be able to put pressure on the insurance carrier to get the claim approved.

After your initial request results in a denial, you should appeal this decision. The denial letter will include the steps you need to take if you disagree with the decision. Typically you have two written appeals and one in-person or over-the-phone appeal. For the first appeal, put together a packet of information for the insurance company that includes supporting documentation to combat the insurance company's reason for denial. This documentation should include letters from all care providers (physicians, dentists, and so on) who are directly involved with your care, indicating that the oral treatment needs are a direct result of the treatment for cancer.

At this point make sure the policy language in your policy booklet is consistent with the insurance company's reason for denial. Insurance companies have been known to deny benefits even though the benefits should be covered as stated in the policy booklet.

Be sure to keep copies of everything you send to your insurance company. Mail the appeal certified mail. Insurance companies "lose" documentation quite often. If your first appeal is not successful, you can submit much of the same information with your second appeal.

Documents should include the following:

■ An appeal letter telling the insurance company why you disagree with its decision and why it should cover your needed dental work. Include factual information and any documented research. Be sure to include all of your identification numbers (policy number, group number, claim number, and so on) in this letter. Request that the denial be reviewed by the insurance company's medical review board (MRB). All insurance companies have MRBs because the expertise of physicians/dentists is needed in special circumstances. The letter should also include a short history of your struggles with oral and head and neck cancer. Finally, include a statement asking the insurance company to overturn its denial and approve your claim.

■ A letter from your dentist and oral specialist addressing specifics of your case.

■ A letter from your medical physician stating that dental issues can be the result of treatment for oral and head and neck cancer.

■ Any important information from your medical records along with copies of similar claims the medical insurance has previously paid.

The next step is to wait for a response from the insurance company. If you get a positive response, celebrate! Make sure that you get this response in writing and that you are aware of any conditions attached to this approval. If the response is negative, appeal to the next level.

Never fail to be optimistic; you must convince the insurance carrier that there is *no doubt* that you *will win* and you will *not stop* until you reach a satisfactory resolution. Make your presence known. Make it a priority to speak to those capable of resolving the issue, or at the very least, have direct access to those with the power to make it happen. Be organized and be prepared! Always let the insurance company know that you may understand their position; however, you *do not agree* with it.

Let them know you are listening but that you expect them to reciprocate and actually *hear* what you are saying. Be pleasant, but *be assertive*. Remind them of their own children and grandchildren; believe it or not, they are people just like us. Be committed because this will take time and endless energy. Believe in yourself and know the result will be worth the many hours of effort, frustration, anger, resentment, and anxiety you have experienced.

Useful Tips

■ Follow up all phone calls with a letter stating what was talked about so that you have a written record.

■ Don't send more information than is asked for.

■ Look for flaws in the denial language.

- Get the insurance company mission statement and use it against the company.
- Challenge everything.
- Appeal to the highest level.
- Request a specialist.
- Inform the insurance company of other medical problems related to oral and head and neck cancer that it has paid for (dermatologist, ENT, and so on).
- Don't give up.
- File your claim on a medical claim form, not a dental claim form.
- Find out the medical diagnosis codes for your particular situation.

C. EVERYTHING YOU NEED TO KNOW ABOUT OBTAINING SOCIAL SECURITY DISABILITY BENEFITS

Scott E. Davis, Disability Attorney

If you have paid taxes to the federal government, part of these taxes purchased a disability policy from the Social Security Administration (SSA). Everyone understands they are entitled to *retirement* benefits from SSA, but many people do not understand they also have *disability* insurance through SSA. Many people mistakenly believe by seeking disability benefits they are "living off the government" if they file a disability claim and receive benefits. It is important to move quickly past this erroneous belief because SSA sold all of us a disability policy and "you better use it" or you may lose it.

Receiving disability benefits from SSA plays an important role in your recovery because it eases the considerable stress that results when and if you are unable to work because of your medical condition.

Not Filing a Claim Brings Devastating Financial Consequences

Unfortunately, not filing a disability claim with SSA when you should brings devastating financial consequences. Many reasons exist to file, foremost that filing a claim protects your earnings record for retirement. Your SSA retirement benefit is based on annual earnings; if you are disabled and not paying social security taxes, then "zeroes" are posted each year to your SSA earnings record. If you are disabled but *do not* file a disability claim, SSA does not know you are disabled and assumes you decided to stop working. SSA then includes the nonearning disability years to your overall earnings record, which potentially reduces your retirement benefit significantly because your SSA earnings record was not protected during the time you were disabled.

A major benefit of being found disabled by SSA is that it protects your earnings record. Beginning with the year you are found disabled, SSA protects your record by not adding in any of the nonearning years when calculating your retirement benefit. The result is if you remain disabled through retirement age, there is no reduction between your disability and retirement benefit.

How Does SSA Define Disability?

SSA's definition of disability is easier to meet than most people realize. Many people mistakenly believe you need a catastrophic injury or need to be confined to a wheelchair or be "permanently" disabled to be eligible. These misconceptions are the reasons that many people do not file a claim, erroneously believing their medical condition is not severe enough to qualify for benefits. Simply put, you qualify for disability benefits if, as a result of any physical or psychological medical condition (or both), you are unable to work in any occupation for a minimum of 12 consecutive months, *or* your condition is expected to result in death.

As long as you or your doctors expect that you will be unable to work in any occupation for *at least 12 months*, then you're eligible for benefits. Permanent disability is not required. Many cancer patients are or can be disabled for several years, receive benefits while recovering from residual effects of treatment, and then eventually return to work.

When to File a Claim

File your claim as soon as you or your doctors believe you meet SSA's definition of disability. If your diagnosis is not treatable and is expected to result in death, immediately file your claim and send the information supporting the diagnosis (i.e., pathology reports, lab results, medical records with clinical findings, and so on) to SSA. Be sure to tell SSA personnel of your condition and ask them to declare your case a "TERI" case. TERI stands for "terminal illness." A TERI case receives expedited claim processing. However, it will be up to you to bring the severity of your condition to SSA's attention; don't assume SSA will do anything.

If your condition is treatable, you might want to continue working as long as you can while receiving treatment because many people find it therapeutic. However, if side effects or residual effects of treatment begin to significantly affect your ability to work on a consistent, daily basis or have an adverse impact on your prognosis, you should file your claim once you have stopped working and expect to be unable to work for a minimum of 12 consecutive months.

At the Latest, File Your Disability Claim Within 5 Years of Being Disabled

You become insured for SSA disability benefits by paying social security taxes for at least 5 of the 10 years *before becoming disabled*. It is critical to understand that SSA's disability insurance does not last forever—you must use it or you eventually lose it. To avoid losing your insurance, be sure to file your claim within 5 years of becoming disabled. File your claim by calling Social Security at 800-772-1213, visiting a local office, or going online at http://www. ssa.gov. There is no charge to file a claim.

Benefits You Will Receive

In addition to protecting your earnings record for retirement, you will receive a monthly monetary payment that varies based on your SSA earnings record. You will also receive Medicare health insurance 29 months after you are first eligible for benefits.

Appeal If Your Claim Is Denied

It is *critical* to appeal if SSA denies your claim. Many people mistakenly believe SSA represents them and will assist in the approval of their claim. The truth is SSA initially denies significantly more claims than it approves. With regard to cancer claims, SSA frequently views *any* initial positive responses to treatment to mean the person can work or return to work. SSA also routinely ignores the residual effects of treatment, preferring instead to focus on response and stage of disease.

Incredibly, SSA statistics confirm that 50% of the time people never appeal the initial denial of their claim. Please avoid becoming a statistic by appealing every denial within 60 days of the date stamped on the denial. It is also critical to not lose hope because eventually the overwhelming majority of claims are approved.

How Social Security Evaluates Head And Neck Cancer

There are several ways SSA can approve a disability claim based on head and neck cancer.

1. **Based on severity of the disease.** Your claim can be approved based solely on the diagnosis depending on the stage of disease. Head and neck cancer falls under Social Security's "Listed Impairments," meaning the law requires your claim to be approved if the stage of disease meets the listed criteria. The specific Adult Listing 13.02 for soft tissue tumors of the head and neck (except salivary glands and thyroid gland, which are listed separately elsewhere) includes the following disease criteria ("Disability Evaluation," 2006):

    A. Inoperable or unresectable.
    B. Persistent disease following initial multimodal antineoplastic therapy.
    C. Recurrent disease following initial anti-neoplastic therapy, except local vocal cord recurrence.
    D. With metastases beyond the regional lymph nodes.
    E. Soft tissue tumors of the head and neck not addressed in A-D, with multimodal antineoplastic therapy. Consider under a disability until at least 18 months from the date of diagnosis. Thereafter, evaluate any residual impairment(s) under the criteria for the affected body system.

If the stage of your disease meets any of these criteria, SSA *must* approve your claim.

2. **Based on inability to sustain work.** What if your condition does not meet SSA's listed criteria? If your diagnosis does not meet the criteria, you can still be approved for disability benefits. Most cancer diagnoses will not initially meet SSA's listed criteria because the listed criteria represent an advanced stage of disease. You are eligible for benefits if you have significant residual effects from cancer treatment or have other medical conditions in addition to the cancer that contribute to your inability to work.

As a general rule, if you do not meet SSA's listed criteria, you must be unable to sustain *sedentary* work on a regular and continuous basis (i.e., SSA defines this as 8 hours per day, 5 days per week) to be eligible. Claims that are based on cancer are often approved because individuals are unable to sustain work due to the cumulative effects of treatment even though the stage of their disease is not advanced enough to meet SSA's listed criteria.

For example, after undergoing radiation and/or chemotherapy, a person's physical and mental stamina can be significantly diminished. Also, the *desire* to communicate and the ability to effectively deal with any stress can be significantly reduced, making consistent work impossible. Furthermore, taking high-dose narcotics for pain control can cause exhaustion and cognitive dysfunction, which further erode stamina and the ability to attend and concentrate.

Because the cumulative effects of cancer treatment can pose significant work limitations, the prudent course is to file your disability claim *sooner rather than later*. When should you file your disability claim? You should do so either when (a) you meet SSA's listed criteria as set forth previously, or (b) you do not meet the criteria but you or your doctors believe you will be unable to sustain full-time work for a minimum of 12 months. Remember, if you are able to return to work after treatment, you can always tell SSA you seek benefits only for the period of time you were off work as long as it lasted more than 12 months, or withdraw your claim altogether if you return to work within 12 months of your initial disability.

Remember to Consider Other Diagnoses That May Preclude Work

Following a cancer diagnosis or after beginning treatment, depression and anxiety may pose significant problems in returning to work. Depression and anxiety, alone or in combination with other limitations resulting from cancer, can be disabling. An example would be a person who has developed significant secondary psychological problems even though that person's cancer treatment appears to have been successful.

Also, if you have undergone invasive oral surgery and are unable to consistently use your voice (or cannot communicate easily), need special accommodations (i.e., a feeding tube), or must take strong narcotics for pain control, you should be eligible for disability benefits.

Hire an Attorney Who Specializes in Social Security Law

SSA's own statistics (Attorney Fee Payment, 2001) prove that one way to significantly increase the odds of obtaining disability benefits is by hiring an experienced social security disability attorney. Consult with and hire an attorney as soon as you believe you may not be able to continue working. Social security attorneys work on a contingency fee, meaning you pay a fee only if your claim is approved and you receive monetary benefits. The attorney should be experienced in social security law because the area is complex and it is easy to make costly mistakes.

Attorney's fees in social security cases are regulated by federal law and almost every attorney uses a standard fee agreement in which the fee is 25% of all past due monetary benefits or $5,300, whichever is the lesser amount. For example, if you have $10,000 in past due benefits when the claim is approved, the fee is $2,500; if you have $40,000 in past due benefits, the maximum fee you pay is $5,300.

An attorney will work directly with SSA personnel so you do not have to. This allows you to focus on recovery. An attorney should also help you complete SSA's forms and will develop medical evidence from your physicians regarding whether you meet SSA's listed criteria. An attorney knows the specific work limitations that are important to obtain from your physician to help prove you are unable to work. SSA generally does not obtain this critical evidence; it simply processes your case and evaluates your ability to work based solely on your medical records.

The following list includes resources for additional information if you are considering applying for disability insurance.

- ■ http://www.scottdavispc.com: Web site of the author where you can find many practical articles concerning disability benefits
- ■ http://www.ssa.gov: Web site of the Social Security Administration
- ■ http://www.nosscr.org: Web site of the National Organization of Social Security Claimants' Representatives from which you can obtain a referral to an experienced social security disability attorney
- ■ http://www.severe.net: Web site of Social Security Disability Benefits Law Information and Resources (Severe.net), hosted by experienced social security attorneys with a wealth of disability information and links to resources

In summary, all people who have paid taxes to the federal government are eligible for retirement benefits and disability insurance. The information provided here is intended to serve as a guide to help you avoid mistakes in seeking disability benefits and help you find the information you need. It is of utmost importance that you not become discouraged during the process of seeking disability benefits and that you follow through with persistence, keeping your spirits high while fighting for the benefits for which you are entitled.

References

Attorney Fee Payment System Improvement Act 2001, Cong. Rec., November 16, 2001 (testimony of Honorable Robert T. Matsui and Honorable E. Clay Shaw).

Disability evaluation under social security. (2006, June). *Blue book.* Available at http://www.ssa.gov/disability/professionals/bluebook

10

MEETING THE CHALLENGES OF CLINICAL TRIALS

A. CLINICAL TRIALS

Nancy E. Leupold, MA

Adapted from the National Cancer Institute's
Educational Materials About Clinical Trials

Clinical trials, also called research studies, test new treatments in people with cancer. The goal of this research is to find better methods to treat cancer and help cancer patients. Clinical trials seek to answer specific scientific questions to find better ways to prevent, detect, and treat diseases and to improve care for people with diseases. Clinical trials may test many types of treatment such as new drugs, new approaches to surgery or radiation therapy, new combinations of treatments, or new methods such as gene therapy. A clinical trial is one of the final stages of a long and careful research process. The search for new treatments begins in the laboratory, where scientists first develop and test new ideas. If an approach seems promising, the next step may be testing a treatment in animals to see how it affects cancer in a living being and whether it has harmful effects. Of course, treatments that work well in the lab or in animals do not always work well in people. Studies are done with cancer patients to find out whether promising treatments are safe and effective.

Types of Clinical Trials

There are several different types of cancer clinical trials. Each type of trial is designed to answer different research questions.

- **Prevention trials** test new approaches, such as medicines, vitamins, minerals, or other supplements that doctors believe may lower the risk of a certain type of cancer. These trials are designed to find the best way to prevent cancer in people who have never had cancer or to prevent cancer from coming back or a new cancer occurring in people who have already had cancer.

- **Screening trials** are designed to find the best way to detect cancer in its early stages, before symptoms develop. These trials involve people who do not have any symptoms of cancer.

- **Diagnostic trials** study tests or procedures that could be used to identify cancer more accurately. Diagnostic trials usually include people who have signs or symptoms of cancer.

■ **Treatment trials** are conducted with people who have cancer. They test new treatments such as a new cancer drug, new approaches to surgery or radiation therapy, new combinations of treatments, or new methods such as gene therapy. These trials are designed to find out what new treatment approaches can help people who have cancer and what the most effective treatment is for people who have cancer.

■ **Quality of life trials** (also called supportive care trials) are designed to explore ways to improve comfort and quality of life for people who have cancer. These trials may study ways to help people who are experiencing side effects from cancer or its treatment.

■ **Genetics studies** are sometimes part of another cancer clinical trial. The genetics component of the trial may focus on how genetic makeup can affect detection, diagnosis, or response to cancer treatment. Population- and family-based genetic research studies differ from traditional cancer clinical trials. In these studies, researchers look at tissue or blood samples, generally from families or large groups of people, to find genetic changes that are associated with cancer. People who participate in genetics studies may or may not have cancer, depending on the study. The goal of these studies is to help understand the role of genes in the development of cancer.

How Patients Are Protected

Clinical trials are conducted in doctors' offices, cancer centers, other medical centers, community hospitals and clinics, and veterans' and military hospitals in cities and towns across the United States and in other countries. Clinical trials may include participants at one or two highly specialized centers, or they may involve hundreds of locations at the same time.

Doctors, nurses, social workers, and other health professionals are part of the treatment team. They will monitor the patient's progress closely. Patients may have more tests and doctor visits than if they were not taking part in a study. Each patient will follow a treatment plan prescribed by the doctor. Patients may also have other responsibilities such as keeping a log or filling out forms about their health. Some studies continue to check on patients even after their treatment is over.

In clinical trials, both research concerns and patient well-being are important. To help protect patients and produce sound results, research with people is carried out according to strict scientific and ethical principles, which include the following:

■ **Each clinical trial has an action plan (protocol) that explains how it will work.**
The study's investigator, usually a doctor, prepares an action plan for the study. Known as a protocol, this plan explains what will be done in the study and why. It outlines how many people will take part in the study, what medical tests they will receive and how often, and the treatment plan. Each doctor who takes part uses the same protocol. For patient safety, each protocol must be approved by the organization that sponsors the study (such as the National Cancer Institute) and the Institutional Review Board (IRB) at each hospital or other study site. This board, which includes consumers, clergy, and health professionals, reviews the protocol to be sure that the research will not expose patients to extreme or unethical risks.

■ **Each study enrolls people who are alike in key ways.**
Each study's protocol describes the characteristics that all patients in the study must have. Called eligibility criteria, these guidelines differ from study to study, depending on the research purpose. They may include age, gender, the type and stage of cancer, and whether cancer patients who have had prior cancer treatment or who have other health problems can take part.
Using eligibility criteria is an important principle of medical research that helps produce reliable results. During a study, they help protect patient safety so that people who are likely to be harmed by study drugs or other treatments are not exposed to the risk. After results are in, they also help doctors know which

patient groups will benefit if the new treatment being studied is proved to work. For instance, a new treatment may work for one type of cancer but not for another, or it may be more effective for men than women.

■ **The informed consent process is an integral part of research.**

Informed consent, a legal, regulatory, and ethical concept, is the process of learning the key facts about a clinical trial before deciding whether to participate. It is also a continuing process throughout the study to provide information for participants. To help someone decide whether or not to participate, the doctors and nurses involved in the trial explain the details of the study. If the participant's native language is not English, translation assistance can be provided. Then the research team provides an informed consent document that includes details about the study, such as its purpose, duration, required procedures, and key contacts. Risks and potential benefits are explained in this document. The participant then decides whether or not to sign the document. The process does not end with the signing of informed consent documents. If new benefits, risks, or side effects are discovered during the trial, researchers must inform participants. Informed consent is not a contract, and the participant may withdraw from the trial at any time. Participants are encouraged to ask questions at any time.

Cancer clinical trials are usually conducted in a series of steps, called *phases*. Treatment clinical trials are always assigned a phase. However, screening, prevention, diagnostic, and quality-of-life studies do not always have a phase nor do genetics clinical trials.

Each phase answers different questions about the new treatment.

■ *Phase I* trials are the first step in testing a new treatment in humans. In these studies, researchers look for the best way to give a new treatment (e.g., by mouth, IV drip, or injection and number of times a day). They also try to find out if and how the treatment can be given safely (e.g., best dose), and they watch for any harmful side effects. Because less is known about the possible risks and benefits in phase I, these studies usually include only a limited number of patients, between 15 and 30, who would not be helped by other known treatments.

▨ *Phase II* trials continue to test the safety of the new agent and begin to evaluate how well it works against a specific type of cancer. As in phase I, only a small number of people (fewer than 100) take part. In general, these participants have been treated with chemotherapy, surgery, or radiation, but treatment has not been effective. It is important to remember that when a phase II trial begins, it is not yet known if the agent tested works against the specific cancer being studied. Unpredictable side effects can also occur in these trials.

▨ *Phase III* trials focus on how a new treatment compares with standard treatment (treatment currently accepted and most widely used). Researchers want to learn whether the new treatment is better than, the same as, or worse than the standard treatment. They assign patients by chance either to a group taking the new treatment (called the treatment group) or to a group taking standard treatment (called the control group). This method, called randomization, helps avoid bias (having the study's results affected by human choices or other factors not related to the treatments being tested).

Comparing similar groups of people taking different treatments for the same type of cancer is another way to make sure that study results are real and caused by the treatment rather than by chance or other factors. Comparing treatments with each other often shows clearly which one is more effective or has fewer side effects.

In most cases, studies move into phase III testing only after a treatment shows promise in phases I and II. Phase III trials may include hundreds to thousands of people around the country (and world) ranging from people newly diagnosed with cancer to people with extensive disease.

▨ *Phase IV* trials are used to further evaluate the long-term safety and effectiveness of a treatment. Less common than phase I, II, and III trials, phase IV trials usually take place after the new treatment has been approved for standard use.

Benefits and Risks of
Participating in a Clinical Trial

While a clinical trial is a good choice for some people, this treatment option has possible benefits and drawbacks.

Possible Benefits

■ Clinical trials offer high-quality (high-quality is somewhat subjective) cancer care.

■ Participants receive regular and careful medical attention from a research team that includes doctors and other health professionals.

■ Participants have access to promising new approaches that are often not available outside the clinical trial setting.

■ The approach being studied may be more effective than the standard approach.

■ Participants may be the first to benefit from the new method under study.

■ Results from the study may help others in the future.

Possible Drawbacks

■ New drugs or procedures under study are not always better than, or even as good as, standard care.

■ New treatments may have side effects that doctors do not expect or that are worse than those of standard treatment

■ Participants in randomized trials will not be able to choose the approach they receive.

■ Even standard treatments, proved effective for many people, do not help everyone.

■ Health insurance and managed care providers do not always cover all patient care costs in a study.

■ The protocol may require more time and attention than would a nonprotocol treatment, including trips to the study site, more treatments, hospital stays, or complex dosage requirements.

To find answers to questions about how clinical trials work and patients' rights and protections, consult a doctor, nurse, or other health care professional.

Where to Find Information About Clinical Trials

■ **NCI-sponsored clinical trial programs:** http://www.nci.nih. gov/clinical_trials

■ **National Institute of Health (NIH) clinical trials:** http:// www.clinicaltrials.gov

■ **National Cancer Institute Clinical Trials Education Series:** http://www.cancer.gov/clinicaltrials/learning/clinical-trials-education-series

■ The **National Library of Medicine's Web site** offers links to resources for finding the results of clinical trials. It includes information about published and unpublished results. http://www. nlm.nih.gov/services/ctresults.html

■ **NCI's PDQ (Physician Data Query)** clinical trials registry can be searched using a basic search form that allows selection of a type of cancer, stage/subtype, type of trial, and location. It is also possible to search for trials using additional criteria such as type of treatment/intervention, drug name, phase of trial, or a combination of these and other variables by using an advanced search form. Help links at the top of each clinical trials search form lead to more information and tips about searching for clinical trials. http://www.cancer.gov/cancertopics/pdq/cancerdatabase# clinical_trial

■ **TrialCheck** is a search tool developed and maintained by the Coalition of Cancer Cooperative Groups. It consists of groups of doctors and other health professionals that carry out many of the larger cancer clinical trials in the United States that are funded by the National Cancer Institute. This search tool uses nine simple questions. After patients answer these questions, they will receive a list of cancer clinical trials in which they may be eligible to enroll. Trialcheck also allows a patient to search for a cancer clinical trial at specific locations. http://www.trial check.org

■ **EmergingMed** is a free and confidential cancer clinical trial matching and referral service. Patients and caregivers can find matches to clinical trials by calling toll free to speak with patient support specialists (877-601-8601) or by visiting the Emerging-Med Web site. Patients will be encouraged to identify their clinical trial options and then review them with their doctor whenever a treatment decision is necessary. EmergingMed's patient support specialists are available Monday through Friday, 8:30 AM to 6:00 PM ET (except holidays). http://www.emergingmed.com

Costs Associated With a Clinical Trial

Health insurance and managed care providers often do not cover the patient care costs associated with a clinical trial. What they cover varies by health plan and by study. Some health plans do not cover clinical trials if they consider the approach being studied "experimental" or "investigational." However, if enough data show that the approach is safe and effective, a health plan may consider the approach "established" and cover some or all of the costs.

Participants may have difficulty obtaining coverage for costs associated with prevention and screening clinical trials; health plans are currently less likely to have review processes in place for these studies. It may, therefore, be more difficult to get coverage for the costs associated with them. In many cases, it helps to have someone from the research team talk about coverage with representatives of the health plan.

Health plans may specify other criteria that a trial must meet to be covered. The trial might have to be sponsored by a specified organization, be judged "medically necessary" by the health plan, not be significantly more expensive than treatments the health plan considers standard, or focus on types of cancer for which no standard treatments are available. In addition, the facility and medical staff might have to meet the plan's qualifications for conducting certain procedures, such as bone marrow transplants. More information about insurance coverage can be found on the NCI's *Clinical Trials and Insurance Coverage: A Resource Guide* Web page at http://www.cancer.gov/clinicaltrials/learning/insurance-coverage.

Many states have passed legislation or developed policies requiring health plans to cover the costs of certain clinical trials. For more information, visit the NCI's Web site at http://www.cancer.gov/clinicaltrials/developments/laws-about-clinical-trial-costs.

Federal programs that help pay the costs of care in a clinical trial include the following:

- Medicare reimburses patient care costs for its beneficiaries who participate in clinical trials designed to diagnose or treat cancer. Information about Medicare coverage of clinical trials is available at http://www.medicare.gov, or by calling Medicare's toll-free number for beneficiaries at 800-633-4227 (800-MEDICARE). The toll-free number for the hearing impaired is 877-486-2048. Also, the NCI fact sheet *More Choices in Cancer Care: Information for Beneficiaries on Medicare Coverage of Cancer Clinical Trials* is available at http://www.cancer.gov/cancertopics/fact sheet/support/medicare.

- Beneficiaries of TRICARE, the Department of Defense's health program, can be reimbursed for the medical costs of participation in NCI-sponsored phase II and phase III cancer prevention (including screening and early detection) and treatment trials. Additional information is available in the NCI fact sheet *TRICARE Beneficiaries Can Enter Clinical Trials for Cancer Prevention and Treatment Through a Department of Defense and National Cancer Institute Agreement*. This fact sheet can be found at http://www.cancer.gov/cancertopics/factsheet/NCI/TRICARE.

- The Department of Veterans Affairs (VA) allows eligible veterans to participate in NCI-sponsored prevention, diagnosis, and treatment studies nationwide. All phases and types of NCI-sponsored trials are included. The NCI fact sheet *The NCI/VA Agreement on Clinical Trials: Questions and Answers* has more information. It is available at http://www.cancer.gov/cancertopics/fact sheet/NCI/VA-clinical-trials.

Completion of a Clinical Trial

After a clinical trial is completed, the researchers look carefully at the data collected during the trial before making decisions about the meaning of the findings and further testing. After a phase I or II trial, the researchers decide whether to move on to the next phase, or stop testing the agent or intervention because it was not safe or effective. When a phase III trial is completed, the researchers look at the data and decide whether the results have medical importance.

The results of clinical trials are often published in peer-reviewed, scientific journals. Peer review is a process by which experts review the report before it is published to make sure the analysis and conclusions are sound. If the results are particularly important, they may be featured by the media and discussed at scientific meetings and by patient advocacy groups before they are published. Once a new approach has proved safe and effective in a clinical trial, it may become standard practice (standard practice is a currently accepted and widely used approach).

B. FINDING A CLINICAL TRIAL TO MEET YOUR SPECIFIC NEEDS

Patty Delaney

Finding a clinical trial to meet the specific needs of a patient can be a challenge. Unfortunately, there are many formidable barriers that impede patient access to cancer clinical trials. Physicians may be resistant to referring patients to clinical trials, and health insurance may not always cover expenses incurred during participation in a clinical trial. There may be restrictions on eligibility that prohibit participation in a trial, or an individual who is interested in participating in a study may be concerned about receiving a placebo and not the drug being tested. In addition, individuals may have fears about being randomized to receive a treatment that is perceived to be less aggressive than the new unproven treatment. Lastly, individuals may have difficulty locating a trial that meets their needs and may find a daunting challenge in contacting trial sites to learn about the trial status and their eligibility.

The Internet has made a huge difference in improving access to information on cancer clinical trials. The Internet provides sources of information about cancer clinical trials being conducted by a variety of institutions and individuals, including hospitals, drug companies, private doctors, and the government. However, there is no central registry that lists *all* cancer clinical trials.

The passage of the Food and Drug Administration Modernization Act of 1997 (FDAMA) directed the Secretary of Health and Human Services, acting through the Director of National Institutes of Health (NIH), to establish, maintain, and operate a data bank of information on clinical trials for drugs to treat serious or life-threatening diseases and conditions. This database was intended to be a central resource, providing current information on clinical trials to individuals, other members of the public, and health care providers and researchers.

The National Institutes of Health (NIH), through its National Library of Medicine (NLM) and with input from the FDA and others, developed the Clinical Trials Data Bank at http://www.clinical trials.gov. The first version of this data bank was made available to the public on February 29, 2000, on the Internet. At that time, the data bank included primarily NIH-sponsored trials. In March of the same year, the FDA issued guidelines to members of the pharmaceutical industry that outlined when and how they were to list their trials on the government clinicaltrials.gov Web site. When the sponsor of a clinical trial begins to investigate whether its drug is effective (phase II, III, and IV clinical trials) in serious and life-threatening diseases and conditions, the trial's sponsor, including drug companies, academic medical centers, or individual doctors, must list that phase II, III, or IV trial in http://www.clinical trials.gov. The trial sponsors must list the following information:

- Purpose of the trial
- Patient eligibility criteria
- Location of the trial sites
- Phone number and name of a contact person

Unfortunately, not all cancer clinical trials being conducted by pharmaceutical companies and academic medical centers are listed in clinicaltrials.gov nor are they listed in the National Cancer Institute's trial directory at http://www.cancer.gov. The FDA and cancer patient advocates have been working together to encourage members of the pharmaceutical industry to list their cancer trials as the law requires them to do. Clinicaltrials.gov presently lists *all* cancer clinical trials being conducted by the NIH, which includes National Cancer Institute trials and also trials supported by pharmaceutical companies. Some cancer experts estimate that approximately 60% to 70% of cancer trials are supported by the pharmaceutical companies. Unfortunately, not all of these trials are listed on http://www.clinicaltrials.gov.

Some new cancer drugs and biologics that are being developed by pharmaceutical companies are listed in a publication every 2 years by the Pharmaceutical Research and Manufacturers of America (PhRMA), the pharmaceutical companies' trade association. These cancer trials conducted by pharmaceutical companies can also be found on the PhRMA Web site at http://www.phrma.org. Regrettably, this, too, is not a comprehensive list of cancer clinical trials. Other sources for clinical trials include newspaper articles, medical journals, not-for-profit and for-profit Web sites as well as the Web sites of individual pharmaceutical companies.

With so much information available, how does one find the latest drugs being studied specifically for oral and head and neck cancer?

Following are some sources of information that may be help-ful in finding a clinical trial to fit a patient's needs.

- **National Institutes of Health (NIH) Web site: http://www. clinicaltrials.gov**. The fact that this clinical trials Web site exists at all is due exclusively to the patient advocacy community, espe-cially cancer patient advocates. The patient advocates lobbied Congress to make it a requirement that drug companies add their clinical trials of drugs for serious and life-threatening diseases and conditions to a publicly accessible database as soon as the drug companies begin to investigate the effectiveness of their unapproved drug. Investigations of a drug's effectiveness usually begin at phase II after the phase I trials have been completed.

- **National Cancer Institute's (NCI) Web site: http://www. cancer.gov/clinicaltrials**. The NCI clinical trial database can be searched by selecting a specific cancer from a list on its Web site. NCI also maintains a valuable clinical trial telephone serv-ice. It can also be accessed by telephone at 800-4-CANCER.

- **American Cancer Society's (ACS) Web site: http://www. cancer.org**. This site provides a confidential matching service for clinical trials nationwide as well as other clinical trial infor-mation. To access the Web page, search for "clinical trials."

- **Support for People with Oral and Head and Neck Cancer (SPOHNC) Web site: http://www.spohnc.org**. This site pro-vides access to clinical trials information. Select "Clinical Trials" under Cancer Information on the home page. The clinical trials listed on this Web site are those related to oral and head and neck cancer. On this Web page, you will find different types of clinical trials, what happens in them, the clinical trial process, information on clinical trial phases, and more.

- **Pharmaceutical Research and Manufacturers of America (PhRMA) Web site: http://www.phrma.org**. This site has clinical trials information listed under the tab Medicines In Development. This Web site is the drug industry's trade associa-tion. It lists new drugs that are in development and the name of the company developing the drug.

■ **Coalition of Cancer Cooperative Groups (CCCG) Web site: http://www.cancertrialshelp.org**. The Coalition of Cancer Cooperative Groups is the nation's premier network of cancer clinical trials specialists. Its diverse, comprehensive membership includes all 10 of the nation's federally funded cancer Cooperative Groups, cancer centers, academic medical centers, community hospitals, physicians, and more than 40 patient advocacy groups.

While the Internet is a valuable resource, it is often not interactive. For example, if the information in the clinical trial listing is unclear, it may not be possible to have your specific questions answered online and in a timely manner. However, a phone number is usually included in the clinical trial listing, and you may be able to get answers to specific questions about a given trial by calling the number listed.

Researching a Clinical Trial That Is Right for You

Before deciding on a specific clinical trial to meet your needs, you should take the following steps to understand your diagnosis, treatment options, and the trials that may be available to you.

Step 1. Learn as much about your disease and diagnosis as you possibly can—for example, the specific type of cancer, the stage of the disease, the size of the tumor, the cell type, the tumor locations, and the standard treatment for your diagnosis. If the diagnosis is a recurrence, you should have a record available of your previous treatment, including the drug names, dates of treatment and the number of treatments, and the location and extent of the recurrence.

Step 2. Write down your diagnosis and treatment information or type it into a computer and keep it accessible in a file you can easily consult. Remember to always have this information with you when you are inquiring about a clinical trial. Practice reporting a summary of your diagnosis with a relative or friend. You should be able to recount your diagnosis in a few minutes, similar to the way one doctor might report your diagnosis to another doctor, with no extraneous information, just the facts. For example: "I was 50 years old when I was diagnosed with stage III squamous cell carcinoma of the base of the tongue. I had 36 external beam radiation therapy treatments coupled with weekly chemotherapy. The tumor on my tongue shrunk and what remained was surgically removed along with some malignant lymph nodes. It is now a year and a half since my surgery, and I have just been diagnosed with a recurrence of the cancer. I am now looking for a clinical trial."

Step 3. Ask your doctor's staff for assistance if you are uncertain about the details of your diagnosis. Remember that information in your medical record can easily be obtained by the staff in your doctor's office. You do not have to take your doctor's time to make this request.

Step 4. Let your doctor know you are investigating clinical trial options. Physicians, especially oncologists, are extremely busy and may not have the time or staff available to explore this option with you. However, your doctor should know that you are pursuing this option and that you welcome his or her advice while you are in the information-gathering phase.

Step 5. Visit the Web sites listed previously to review the information on the trials that interest you. Each trial that is listed will usually have the following components: the trial objective, in other words, what the scientists are trying to learn from conducting the trial; where the trial will be conducted; and the patient eligibility criteria. Patient eligibility criteria are used to select which patients will be in the trial; examples of criteria are age, extent of disease involvement, or the amount of prior treatment the patient has received.

Step 6. Compare the trial eligibility criteria you found on the Web page or discussed with a clinical trial telephone service with your diagnosis and then select the trials you think might be a match. Review these trials with your doctor, your family, and head and neck cancer survivors to get their opinions.

Before you seek your doctor's advice, try to narrow the selection down to two or three trials. It is important to avoid presenting your doctor with a huge stack of trials. If you need help in narrowing the choice, patient advocacy organizations can assist you, or you can call 800-4-CANCER.

Selecting the Trial That Is Right for You

Step 1. Determine how far are you willing to travel from your home to participate in a trial.

Step 2. Locate the phone number of the trial site where you are interested in participating. Sometimes the phone number that is listed is the trial site and sometimes it is an 800 number to a service proofing the trial information to callers. Telephone numbers can be found on the clinical trial listing.

Step 3. Review the trial eligibility criteria. If you think you may be eligible to enter the trial, call the trial site to determine whether you are in fact eligible for the trial. Your doctor can call the trial site for you, but that may not be necessary. At some point, the trial site may want to speak to your doctor, but while you are in the process of gathering information, it is not usually necessary.

Step 4. Ask to speak to the protocol nurse or research assistant when you reach the trial site. The phone number listed for the clinical trial is that of the physician who is also known as the principal investigator of the clinical trial. You are only gathering information, so it is not necessary to speak to this physician. Eventually your doctor will speak to the principal investigator, but only when you decide to enter the trial.

Step 5. Ask the following questions when speaking with the research assistant or protocol nurse:

■ Is the trial still recruiting patients? If the trial is no longer recruiting patients, the rest of the questions are irrelevant. Keep in mind that sometimes the database information lags behind the actual status of a clinical trial. For example, a trial may be listed as open and recruiting patients but may actually have closed and the database has not yet been updated to reflect that fact.

■ Am I eligible for the trial? This is the point when you recount a brief summary of your history, for example, the exact diagnosis, cell type, stage of disease, your age, and so on.

■ What is the objective of the trial?

■ How may patients have been recruited so far? How many more will be recruited?

■ Can I get a copy of the informed consent document?

Step 6. Express your interest in entering the trial if is still recruiting, but consult your family, your physician, and your patient advocacy organization before making your final decision. Remember that there are a many points of view concerning clinical trials. Deciding to participate is your decision.

Following are some additional questions to consider in your decision-making process:

■ Will my health insurance pay for my care if I enter a trial?
■ Should I do it if my doctor disagrees?
■ Will placebos be used and why?
■ What support is offered to patients in the trial? For example, are travel expenses reimbursed?
■ Can I trust Web site information?

Finding a clinical trial to meet your needs is a complex process. However, there are many experienced cancer survivors waiting and willing to help you. The staff at the FDA's Cancer Liaison Program (301-827-4460 or http://www.fda.gov/oashi/cancer/cancer.html) and members of the National Survivor Volunteer Network of SPOHNC are available to assist you.

11

PRODUCTS, THERAPIES, AND SURVIVOR INPUT: RESOURCES FOR COPING WITH THE CHALLENGES OF SIDE EFFECTS OF TREATMENT

Nancy E. Leupold, MA

Oral and head and neck cancer and its treatments can cause various side effects during a survivor's cancer journey. Some of these side effects can be easily controlled; others may require special types of care. The following tables have been compiled to provide information and supportive care to oral and head and neck cancer survivors who may be experiencing side effects of cancer and its treatment. It is important to keep in mind that not all survivors will experience the same side effects and not all suggested resources will be of help to everyone.

For information concerning the challenges of eating and swallowing and nutrition, please see the appropriate chapters in this book.

DISCLAIMER: Support for People with Oral and Head and Neck Cancer (SPOHNC) does not endorse any treatments or products mentioned in this chapter. *It is of utmost importance that you consult with your physician and other health care professionals before using any of the treatments, products, tips, or suggestions presented on the following pages.*

Xerostomia (Dry Mouth) Saliva Substitutes

Product	Source	Description	How to Access
Entertainer's Secret®	KLI Corp.	Moisturizes, soothes, lubricates, mends and protects sensitive mucous membranes of the throat and larynx. A spray for dry sore throat and hoarse voice.	Call 800-308-7452. http://www.entertainers-secret.com
MedOral™ Dry Mouth Treatment	Atos Medical Inc.	Moisturizes and lubricates the oral cavity. Adheres to oral mucosa, providing a smooth slick surface. Nonirritating non-aerosol pump spray.	800-217-0025 http://www.atos.com
Moi-stir Solution®	Kingswood Laboratories	Moisturizes and lubricates oral tissues.	Ask pharmacist to order 800-968-7772.
Mouthkote®	Parnell Pharmaceuticals	Moisturizes mouth. Oral moisturizer with Yerba Santa. Contains xylitol. No sugar or alcohol.	Ask pharmacist to order or call 800-457-4276 http://www.yslabs.com http://www.parnellpharm.org
Numoisyn™ Liquid	Align Pharmaceuticals	Used to replace saliva when salivary glands are damaged. An oral solution with a viscosity similar to that of natural saliva.	**Consult your physician. By prescription only.** 908-834-0960 http://www.alignpharma.com

continues

Xerostomia (Dry Mouth) Saliva Substitutes *continued*

Product	Source	Description	How to Access
Numoisyn™ Lozenges	Align Pharmaceuticals	Increases salivary secretion by stimulating gustatory (taste) pathways. Lozenges.	**Consult your physician. By prescription only.** 908-834-0960 http://www.alignpharma.com
Oasis® Moisturizing Mouthwash	GlaxoSmithKline (GSK)	Moisturizes mouth. Locks in moisture. Protects from dryness.	Pharmacies. 800-777-2500 http://www.oasisdrymouth.com
Oasis® Moisturizing Mouth Spray	GlaxoSmithKline (GSK)	Moisturizes mouth. Locks in moisture. Protects from dryness. Sugar free, alcohol free.	Pharmacies. 800-777-2500 http://www.oasisdrymouth.com
Oral Balance™ Gel	Laclede Professional Products	Soothes and protects oral tissues. Antibacterial moisturizing gel.	Pharmacies. 800-922-5856 http://www.biotene.com
Oral Balance™ Liquid	Laclede Professional Products	Helps promote healing as it moistens. Helpful in relieving severe dry mouth symptoms: burning, sore tissues, cotton palate, and swallowing difficulties.	Pharmacies. 800-922-5856 http://www.biotene.com
Oral Balance™ Spray	Laclede Professional Products	Moisturizes mouth. Soothes and relieves dryness. Contains 5 moisturizers, 18 amino acids, calcium, and omega-3.	Pharmacies. 800-922-5856 http://www.biotene.com

Product	Source	Description	How to Access
Quench® Mist mouth spray	Mueller Sports Medicine Inc.	Moisturizes mouth. Spray. Lemon, orange, cherry and grape flavors.	Sporting goods store 800-356-9522 http://www.quenchgum.com.
Stoppers 4® Dry Mouth Spray	Woodridge Labs Inc.	Moisturizes mouth. Multiple enzyme formulation to maintain optimum moisture levels.	Pharmacies. 888-766-7331 http://www.woodridgelab.com
THAYERS® Dry Mouth Spray	Henry Thayer & Company	Provides saliva-replacing moisture and instant relief from dryness. All natural, sugar-free. Peppermint and Citrus flavors.	Health food stores. Or call 203-226-0940. http://www.thayers.com
Water; a survivor's best friend	Survivor input	Moisturizes the mouth. No sugar or salt. Available in many sizes and containers.	Pharmacies. Supermarkets. Homes.

Xerostomia (Dry Mouth): Products and Therapies to Stimulate Salivary Flow

(Some products for dry mouth may "sting" on contact, but "stinging" usually disappears.)

Product	Distributor	Description	How to Access
Acupuncture	Survivor input	May be helpful in stimulating salivary glands to produce saliva.	Consult your physician. 510-649-8488 http://www.hmieducation.com

continues

Xerostomia (Dry Mouth): Products and Therapies to Stimulate Salivary Flow *continued*

Product	Distributor	Description	How to Access
Biotène™ Dry Mouth Gum	Laclede Professional Products	Stimulates salivary flow. Antibacterial. Sugar free. Reduces mouth sugars. Doesn't stick to dentures.	Pharmacies. 800-922-5856 http://www.biotene.net
Carefree® Koolerz™ Xylitol Gum	The Hershey Company	Helps to stimulate saliva flow. Sweetened with Xylitol available in many flavors.	Pharmacies. Supermarkets. 800-468-1714 http://www.hersheys.com/koolerz
Care*free Sugarless Gum	Nabisco Inc.	Helps to stimulate saliva flow. Sugarless gum. Natural and artificial sweeteners. Assorted flavors.	Pharmacies. Supermarkets. Convenience stores. 312-644-2121
Evoxac® (Cevimeline HCl)	Daiichi Pharmaceuticals	Stimulates salivary glands to produce more saliva. Capsules. Not presently approved for head and neck cancer patients.	**Consult your physician. By prescription only.** http://www.evoxac.com
Extra™ Sugar free Gum	Wm. Wrigley Jr. Company	Stimulates saliva flow. Sugar-free gum sweetened with sorbitol, mannitol, and aspartame. Assorted natural and artificial flavors.	Pharmacies. Supermarkets. Convenience stores. 800-974-4539
Fruit pits: peach, cherry, plum, etc.	Survivor input	Sucking on fruit pit may stimulate salivary flow.	Supermarkets. Farm stands.

Product	Distributor	Description	How to Access
Maxisal™	Amarillo Biosciences Inc.	Promotes oral comfort by helping to stimulate and enhance salivary function. A dietary supplement containing Salive™.	806-376-1741 http://www.amarbio.com
Salagen® (pilocarpine HCL)	MGI Pharma Inc.	Stimulates the salivary glands to increase production of saliva. Tablets. 5 g and 7.5 mg.	**Consult your physician. By prescription only.** 800-562-0679
SalivaSure™	Scandinavian Formulas, Inc.	Helps to increase saliva production and freshen breath. Self-dissolving lozenges.	800-688-2276 http://www. scandinavianformulas.com
THAYERS® Dry Mouth Lozenges	Henry Thayer & Company	Stimulates saliva flow providing relief from dryness. All natural. Sugar free.	Health food stores. 888-842-9371 http://www.thayers.com
TheraGum™	Omnii International	Stimulates saliva flow. Strengthens teeth. May reduce caries. Aids in reducing plaque. Promotes neutral pH. 100% xylitol.	Available in dental offices. http://www.4oralcare.com
Theraspray™	Omnii Oral Pharmaceuticals— 3M ESPE	Stimulates saliva flow to help strengthen teeth. Fights oral malodor. Contains Microdent®, a patented plaque reduction agent. Alcohol-free mouth moistening breath spray with xylitol.	Available in dental offices. http://www.4oralcare.com
Trident™ Gum	Cadbury Adams	Stimulates saliva flow. Flavored, sugarless chewing gum. Many flavors sweetened with xylitol.	Pharmacies. Supermarkets. Convenience stores.

Products to Help With Thick Saliva

Product	Source	Description	How to Access
Adolph's meat tenderizer	Survivor input	May help to break up thick saliva. 1 teaspoon tenderizer in 1 cup water. Swish and gargle but do not swallow. Do not use if there are open lesions in the mouth.	Supermarkets.
Bed wedge	Survivor input	Elevates head and supports the back and torso on a gradual slope. Available in different heights.	Medical supply companies. Online stores.
Blocks of wood under head of bed	Survivor input	Elevates the head.	Home Depot. Lowe's. Local lumberyard.
Ginger tea (decaffeinated)	Survivor input	Sipping ginger tea may help to break up thick saliva.	Health food stores. Online stores.
Mucinex® Tablets (guaifenesin) Time released.	Adams Laboratories Survivor input	Helps loosen phlegm (mucus) and thin bronchial secretions to rid the bronchial passageways of bothersome mucus and make coughs more productive. An expectorant.	**Consult your physician.** Pharmacies. Supermarkets.

Product	Source	Description	How to Access
Papaya juice (100% pure)	Survivor input	Swish and swallow papaya juice from a glass. May help to cut thick saliva. Do not use if there are open lesions in the mouth.	Supermarkets. Health food stores. Online stores.
Papaya juice and club soda or seltzer	Survivor input	Sip slowly from a glass to help cut thick saliva. Do not use if there are open lesions in the mouth	Supermarkets. Convenience stores. Health food stores. Online stores.
Robitussin® (guaifenesin)	Wyeth Consumer Healthcare Survivor input	Helps to thin mucus and makes it easier to cough it up. An expectorant.	Consult your physician Pharmacies. Supermarkets.
Room humidifier (cool mist)	Survivor input	May help to thin secretions. Use to moisten room air, especially at night. Must be routinely cleaned to avoid mold contamination.	Department stores. Pharmacies. Medical supply stores. Online stores.
Seltzer (unflavored)	Survivor input	Sip or gargle and drink to help cut thick saliva.	Supermarkets. Convenience stores.

Products to Soothe the Oral Mucosa

Product	Source	Description	How to Access
Acidophilus	Survivor input	Can help restore normal bacterial flora in the body. May be helpful in the treatment of thrush. Probiotic, also called "friendly bacteria" or "good bacteria." Capsules or liquid.	Health food stores.
Aloe vera juice	Survivor input	Helps with healing mouth sores. Swish; hold in mouth; spit out.	Health food stores.
Caphosol®	Cytogen Corp.	Provides soothing relief of oral throat. A mouth rinse to moisten, lubricate and clean the oral cavity and mucosa of the mouth, tongue and throat.	**Consult your physician. By prescription only.** 800-833-3533
Diflucan® (fluconazole)	Pfizer, Inc.	Used to treat fungal infections, including yeast infections of the mouth, throat, esophagus and other organs. Slows the growth of fungi.	**Consult your physician. By prescription only.** 800-438-1985
GelClair®	EKR Therapeutics	Provides relief of pain from mucositis by adhering to the mucosal surface of the mouth. Soothes oral lesions of various etiologies. A bio-adherent oral gel.	**Consult your physician. By prescription only.**

Product	Source	Description	How to Access
GUM® Chlorhexidine Gluconate Oral Rinse USP, 0.12%	Sunstar Americas Inc.	Helps fight bacteria, viruses, bacterial spores and fungi. Anti-microbial oral rinse. Alcohol free. Therapeutically equivalent to Peridex®.	**Consult your dentist.** 888-777-3101
Gum® Rincinol™ P.R.N.™ Soothing Oral Rinse	Sunstar Americas, Inc.	Forms a protective barrier promoting healing of canker and mouth sores. No numbing benzocaine—No stinging hydrogen peroxide—No burning alcohol!	Pharmacies. 888-777-3101 http://www.drugstore.com
Hurricaine® spray, liquid or gel	Beutlich, LP, Pharmaceuticals	Relieves pain temporarily. Topical anesthetic containing 20% benzocaine. Several flavors.	Pharmacies. 800-238-8542 http://www.beutlich.com
Kefir	Survivor input	Swish & swallow. Pro-biotic dairy product that may restore oral flora.	Health food stores.
Kepivance® (palifermin)	Amgen Oncology Survivor Input	Helps to decrease the incidence and duration of oral mucositis. Palifermin has not yet been approved for head and neck cancer patients.	**Consult your physician. By prescription only.**
Mary's Magic Mouthwash	Survivor input	Helps to relieve oral pain. A compound containing benadryl, an antiseptic, an antibiotic, and pain reliever. Swish and spit.	**Consult your physician. By prescription only.**

continues

Products to Soothe the Oral Mucosa *continued*

Product	Source	Description	How to Access
Mouthwash	Survivor input	Helps relieve pain due to oral ulcerations, Compound of Benadryl® elixir, Maalox®, Mylanta® or Kaopectate. Swish and spit.	**Consult your physician. By prescription only.**
Mouth Rinse (baking soda and salt)	Survivor input	Helps to relieve pain. Mix ½ teaspoon baking powder and ½ teaspoon salt with 1 quart warm water. Swish and spit out. Rinse with water.	**Consult your physician.** Ingredients available at supermarkets.
Mycelex® (clotrimazole)	Ortho-McNeil Pharmaceutical	Used to treat yeast infections of the mouth. Anti-fungal medication.	**Consult your physician. By prescription only.** 800-526-7736
Mycostatin® (nystatin rinse)	Bristol-Myers Squibb Company	Helps to treat thrush/candidiasis. Swish, gargle, spit. Liquid, powder, lozenge.	**Consult your physician. By prescription only.** 800-321-1335
Peridex® (chlorhexidine gluconate, 0.12%)	Omnii Oral Pharmaceuticals— 3M ESPE	Helps to fight bacteria, viruses, bacterial spores and fungi. An antiseptic and disinfectant antimicrobial. May help to prevent candidiasis.	**By prescription only. Dental offices.** 800-643-3639

Product	Source	Description	How to Access
Prevention® Antibacterial Mouth Rinse	Prevention Laboratories, LLC	Fights plaque & gingivitis. Kills bacteria; fights herpes virus & thrush. Helps heal mouth sores. Zinc/Hydrogen Peroxide. Alcohol free formula.	Walgreen's Pharmacy. 800-473-1205 http://www.preventionlab.com
Prevention® Oncology Mouth Rinse	Prevention Laboratories, LLC	Soothes the oral tissues. Helps control sore gums & ulcerated tissue. Controls thrush. Alcohol free.	Walgreen's Pharmacy. 800-473-1205 http://www.preventionlab.com
Sporanox™ (itraconazole)	Ortho-McNeil, Inc.	Used to treat yeast infections of the mouth and throat. Also used to treat fungal infections of the fingernails and/or toenails	**Consult your physician. By prescription only.** 800-526-7736
Spry Rain™ Dry Mouth Spray	Xlear, Inc.	Provides immediate relief to dry mouth conditions with safe and effective xylitol. Has moisturizing effects and encourages increased salivation. Natural spearmint flavor.	Health food stores. 877-599-5327 http://www.xlear.com
Tea tree oil (diluted)	Survivor input	May be helpful for the treatment of thrush. Tea tree oil is known as an effective antiseptic and fungicide. Promotes tissue healing.	**Consult your physician.** Health food stores.

continues

157

Products to Soothe the Oral Mucosa *continued*

Product	Source	Description	How to Access
THAYERS® Slippery Elm Lozenges	Henry Thayer & Company	Soothes the tissues of the mouth and throat. All natural, sugar free lozenges. Several flavors available.	Health food stores. 888-842-9371 http://www.thayers.com
Toothette® Oral Care Mouth Moisturizer	Sage Products, Inc.	Soothes and moisturizes lips and oral tissues with vitamin E and coconut oil.	Ask your pharmacist to order. HDIS Home Care. 800-269-4663 http://www.sageproducts.com
Toothette® Swabs	Sage Products, Inc.	Cleans teeth and soothes mouth. Various swabs available.	Ask your pharmacist to order. HDIS Home Care 800-269-4663 http://www.sageproducts.com
UlcerEase®	Med-Derm Pharmaceuticals	Helps to relieve pain due to mouth ulcers, canker sores and other irritations. Sodium bicarbonate based alcohol-free anesthetic mouth rinse.	Pharmacies. 800-877-8869 http://www.crown laboratories.com http://www.drugstore.com
Xylocaine Viscous® (lidocaine viscous)	AstraZeneca Pharmaceuticals	May help to relieve pain associated with radiation mucositis. Topical anesthetic.	**Consult your physician. By prescription only.** 800-236-9933

Products to Soothe the Nasal Passages

Product	Source	Description	How to Access
Ayr® Saline Nasal Gel Moisturizing Swabs	B.F. Ascher & Co.	Helps moisturize and soothe dry noses.	Pharmacies. Online stores. 913-888-1880 http://www.drugstore.com
Ayr® Saline Nasal Gel with soothing aloe	B.F. Ascher & Co.	Moisturizes and soothes dry, stuffy sore, tender noses.	Pharmacies. Online Stores. 913-888-1880 http://www.drugstore.com
Homemade rinse	Survivor input	Helps relieve stuffiness and blockage. ½ tsp salt, ½ tsp baking soda mixed in warm water. Use nasal irrigator syringe to administer.	**Consult your physician.** Supermarket for ingredients.
NeilMed Sinus Rinse™	NeilMed Pharmaceuticals	Helps relieve stuffiness and blockage of the nasal passages. A therapeutic, saline nasal irrigation & moisturizing system.	Pharmacies. 877-477-8633 http://www.drugstore.com http://www.neilmed.com
Pretz® Concentrate	Parnell Pharmaceuticals	Used for moisturizing the nasal mucosa and sinuses. Preservative free with Yerba Santa and xylitol. Mix with water.	800-457-4276 http://www.parnellpharm.com http://www.yslabs.com
Pretz® Irrigation	Parnell Pharmaceuticals	Provides moisturizing nasal irrigation with natural Yerba Santa.	800-457-4276 http://www.parnellpharm.com http://www.yslabs.com

continues

Products to Soothe the Nasal Passages *continued*

Product	Source	Description	How to Access
Pretz® Spray	Parnell Pharmaceuticals	Used for moisturizing the nasal mucosa and sinuses. 3% glycerin in saline nasal spray with Yerba Santa.	800-457-4276 http://www.parnellpharm.com http://www.yslabs.com

Products to Help Trismus
(A restriction in the opening of the mouth)

Product	Source	Description	How to Access
Botox®	Allergan Inc.	Decreases spasms of jaw muscles. Local injection.	**Consult your physician. By prescription only.** 800-377-7790
Dynasplint® Trismus System	Dynasplint Systems Inc.	Aids in restoring range of motion to tight and short jaw muscles that cause restricted mouth opening.	800-638-6771 http://www.dynasplint.com
TheraBite® Jaw Motion Rehabilitation System™	Atos Medical	Designed to treat trismus, limited jaw mobility and orofacial pain. Utilizes repetitive passive motion and stretching to restore mobility and flexibility of jaw musculature, associated joints, and connective tissues.	Consult insurance company for preauthorization. 877-458-ATOS (2867) or 800-217-0025 http://www.atosdirect.com

Products for Oral Hygiene

Product	Distributor	Description	How to Access
Aquafresh®	GlaxoSmithKline (GSK)	Fluoride toothpaste for cavity protection. Tubes and pumps.	Pharmacies. Supermarkets. 800-897-5623 http://www.aquafresh.com
Biotene™ Dry Mouth Denture Grip	Laclede Professional Products	Formulated to provide a strong, long-lasting and comfortable hold in a dry mouth. Soothes minor irritations. Refreshing taste.	Pharmacies. 800-922-5856 http://www.biotene.net
Biotene™ Dry Mouth Toothpaste	Laclede Professional Products	Contains antibacterial enzymes to destroy bacteria. Helps restore natural antibacterial system present in saliva. Contains fluoride. 4.5 oz. tube.	Pharmacies. 800-922-5856 http://www.biotene.net
Biotene™ Mouthwash	Laclede Professional Products	Breaks down bacteria. Replaces important enzymes. Antibacterial enzyme system. Alcohol free	Pharmacies. 800-922-5856 http://www.biotene.net
Biotene™ PBF Mouthwash	Laclede Professional Products	Formulated to remove and dissolve plaque and biofilm. Alcohol free. Kills germs more effectively. Fresh breath—6× longer	Pharmacies. 800-922-5856 http://www.biotene.net
Biotene™ Super Soft Toothbrush	Laclede Professional Products	Ensures a gentle cleaning without irritating inflamed or unhealthy tissues.	Pharmacies. 800-922-5856 http://www.biotene.net

continues

Products for Oral Hygiene *continued*

Product	Distributor	Description	How to Access
BreathTech Plaque Fighter Spray	Omnii Oral Pharmaceuticals—3M ESPE	Coats, soothes mouth, freshens breath. Daytime plaque fighter to disrupt formation of plaque. Contains xylitol and fluoride. Spray.	**Dental offices.** 800-643-3639
Crest® Complete Extra Soft Toothbrush	Procter & Gamble	Ripple brushes help remove bacterial plaque between teeth and along gum line. Extra soft for gentle brushing.	Pharmacies. Supermarkets. Online stores.
Natural Anti-cavity Fluoride Toothpaste for a Dry Mouth	Toms of Maine®	Aids in the prevention of dental cavities. Contains xylitol. Mild apricot flavor.	Pharmacies. Supermakets. 800-For-Toms http://www.tomsofmaine.com
PerioMed™ Oral Rinse	Omnii Oral Pharmaceuticals—3M ESPE	Contains patented plaque fighter. Alcohol free. Flavored base. Pump.	**Dental offices. By prescription only.** 800-643-3639
Perox-A-Mint®	Sage Products Inc.	Mechanically cleans and debrides with 1.5% hydrogen peroxide.	For information and ordering, 800-269-4663.
Rota-dent® Electric Toothbrush	Pro-Dentec	Power-assisted rotary toothbrush. Soft filament brush tips.	**Dental offices only.** 800-228-5595
Sensodyne® Total Care Toothbrush	GlaxoSmithKline (GSK)	Dome-shaped head designed to adapt to gum line. Extra soft, round-ended bristles to help prevent gum irritation.	Pharmacies. 800-777-2500 http://www.dentist.net

Product	Distributor	Description	How to Access
SmartMouth™ Mouthwash	Triumph Pharmaceuticals	Effective for common and chronic bad breath. 100% alcohol-free, no burning. 2-bottle, 2-pump system.	Pharmacies. Supermarkets. http://www.drugstore.com
SootheRX®	Omnii Oral Pharmaceuticals— 3M ESPE	Indicated for both the rapid and continual relief of dentinal hypersensitivity The first FDA cleared at-home prescription therapy	**Dental Offices.** 800-643-3639 http://www.omniipharma.com

Products to Protect Teeth

Product	Source	Description	How to Access
ACT Rinse® Mouthwash	Johnson & Johnson	Anticavity fluoride rinse (0.05%). Alcohol free and nonirritating. Use once daily after brushing.	Pharmacies.
Custom gel fluoride trays	Dental offices	Used to prevent demineralization of tooth structure and rampant caries. Best way to provide adequate fluoride.	**Consult your dentist.** **Dental offices.**

continues

Products to Protect Teeth *continued*

Product	Source	Description	How to Access
Gel Kam® (0.4% stannous fluoride gel)	Colgate Oral Pharmaceuticals	Provides effective decay prevention.	Pharmacies. 800-468-6502 http://www.colgate.com
Gel-Kam® Home Care Gel	Colgate Oral Pharmaceuticals	Provides sensitivity relief and cavity protection.	Pharmacies. 800-468-6502 http://www.colgate.com
Gel-Kam® Oral Care Rinse	Colgate Oral Pharmaceuticals	Reduces existing plaque. High concentration of stannous fluoride for maximum sensitivity relief.	**Dental offices. By prescription only.** 800-468-6502 http://www.colgate.com
Omnii Gel™ (0.4% stannous fluoride gel)	Omnii Oral Pharmaceuticals—3M ESPE	Provides caries reduction, enhanced remineralization. Brush-on gel. Assorted flavors.	**Dental offices. By prescription only.** 800-643-3639 http://www.omniipharma.com
PerioMed™ (0.63% stannous fluoride oral rinse)	Omnii Oral Pharmaceuticals—3M ESPE	Provides consistent stannous and fluoride ion bioavailability. Contains patented plaque fighter. Alcohol free. Flavored base. Pump.	**Dental offices. By prescription only.** 800-643-3639 http://www.omniipharma.com

Product	Source	Description	How to Access
Phos-Flur® Gel	Colgate Oral Pharmaceuticals	Used frequently with custom mouth trays for daily self-topical use as a dental caries preventative. Promotes remineralization.	**Dental offices. By prescription only.** 800-643-3639 http://www.colgate.com
PreviDent® Brush on Gel	Colgate Oral Pharmaceuticals	Used in a custom mouth tray. Five times the fluoride of over-the-counter toothpastes.	**Dental offices. By prescription only.** 800-643-3639 http://www.colgate.com
PreviDent® Dental Rinse	Colgate Oral Pharmaceuticals	Used as a weekly dental rinse. Four times the fluoride of over-the-counter toothpastes.	**Dental offices. By prescription only.** 800-643-3639 http://www.colgate.com
PreviDent® 5000 Plus toothpaste	Colgate Oral Pharmaceuticals	Used to help prevent cavities. Prescription-strength fluoride treatment	**Dental offices only. By prescription only.** 800-643-3639 http://www.colgate.com
Thera-Flur®-N brand of neutral sodium fluoride gel-drops	Colgate Oral Pharmaceuticals	Helps to prevent dental caries. Once-daily use. Self-applied topical gel for use in custom mouth trays.	**Dental offices. By prescription only.** 800-643-3639 http://www.colgate.com

Products for Radiation Dermatitis

(Check with your radiation oncologist prior to radiation therapy to determine whether skin cream can be used prior to radiation or after radiation, only.)

Product	Source	Description	How to Access
Alra® Therapy Lotion	Neue Cosmetic Company	Developed for the treatment of skin exposed to radiation therapy: Aloe vera gel, lanolin, vitamin E.	877-265-9092 http://www.alra.com http://www.healing baskets.com
Aquaphor® healing ointment	Eucerin Patient input	Reduces healing time. Creates protective barrier that seals in moisture. Helps heal raw, irritated skin caused by radiation treatments.	Pharmacies. Supermarkets. Online drug stores. http://www.eucerinus.com
Biafine®	OrthoNeutrogena, Ortho-McNeil Pharmaceutical	Facilitates the recovery of compromised skin by impacting the three stages of healing. Provides moist environment for healing and repels harmful germs and other external contamination.	**Consult your physician. By prescription only.** 877-738-4624 http://www.orthoneutrogena. com
Burn Blok® After Care Lotion	Medi-Tech International Corp.	Replenishes lost moisture to the skin. Encourages production of collagen fibration. Indicated for management of radiation-induced dermatitis, thermal burns, first- and second-degree burns, sunburn, and rashes.	800-333-0109 http://www.medi-techintl.com http://www.balegoonline.com http://www.amazon.com

Product	Source	Description	How to Access
Elocon® (mometasone furoate)	Schering Corporation	Used to relieve the redness, swelling, itching and discomfort of many skin problems. High potency topical corticosteroid. Cream, ointment, or lotion.	**Consult your physician. By prescription only.** 908-298-4000
Lindi® Body Lotion	Lindi Skin	Helps to improve overall dryness resulting from chemotherapy. Light and refreshing.	800-380-4704 http://www.lindiskin.com
Lindi® Cooler Roll	Lindi Skin	Provides immediate and cooling relief to burned or dehydrated skin. Use *AFTER* each treatment.	800-380-4704 http://www.lindiskin.com
Lindi® Skin Cooler Pad	Lindi Skin	Provides immediate and cooling relief to areas that are burned or dehydrated.	800-380-4704 http://www.lindiskin.com
Mepilex® Border with Safetac® soft silicone technology	Molnlyck Health Care	Used in the management of radiation skin reactions. Pad does not stick to moist wound bed. Absorbs moderate amounts of drainage. Adheres gently to surrounding dry skin.	Online stores. 800-843-8497 http://www.@molnlycke.com
Mepilex® Lite with Safetac® soft silicone technology	Molnlyck Health Care	Used in the management of radiation skin reactions. Thin, flexible, absorbent pad. Maintains a moist wound environment.	Online stores. 800-843-8497 http://www.@molnlycke.com

continues

Products for Radiation Dermatitis *continued*

Product	Source	Description	How to Access
Mepilex® Transfer with Safetac® soft silicone technology	Molnlyck Health Care	Used in the management of radiation skin reactions. A transfer dressing. Pad may be used as a protective layer on minimal or low oozing wounds.	Online stores. 800-843-8497 http://www.@molnlycke.com
MPM CoolMagic® Gel sheets	MPM Medical Inc.	Used to reduce pain from burns and skin reactions to radiation. Allows flow of oxygen. Prevents bacteria and foreign matter from entering the wound.	800-232-5512 http://www.mpmmedicalinc.com 800-461-1370 http://www.suprememedical.com
Polysporin® Ointment	Pfizer	Prevents infection to help speed healing.	Pharmacies. Supermarkets. 800-438-1985
RadiaCream™	Carrington Laboratories	Used for moisturizing skin of radiation patients. Moisturizing cream.	800-358-5205 http://www.carringtonlabs.com
RadiaDres™ Gel Sheet (4" × 4")	Carrington Laboratories	Used in the management of partial thickness wounds relating to radiation-induced dermatitis.	800-358-5205 http://www.carringtonlabs.com
RadiaGel™	Carrington Laboratories	Used before, during, and after radiation. A hydrogel wound dressing with Acemannan Hydrogel™.	**Consult your radiation oncologist. By prescription only.** 800-358-5205 http://www.carringtonlabs.com

Product	Source	Description	How to Access
MPM RadiaPlex®Rx Gel	MPM Medical Inc.	Used to prevent and soothe skin problems associated with radiation dermatitis. A unique combination of complex carbohydrates and hyaluronic acid. Has ability to retain huge quantities of water.	**Consult your radiation oncologist. By prescription only.** 800-232-5512 http://www.mpmmedicalinc.com
Regenecare® Wound Gel	MPM Medical Inc.	Used to reduce rash and itching. Reduces pain from radiation A pain-relieving hydrogel. Contains lidocaine HCl, collagen, and aloe vera.	**Consult your radiation oncologist. By prescription only.** 800-232-5512 http://www.mpmmedicalinc.com
Regenecare® HA Wound Gel	MPM Medical Inc.	Used to reduce rash and itching. Reduces pain from radiation. A pain relieving hydrogel. Contains lidocaine HCl, collagen and aloe vera.	**Consult your radiation oncologist. By prescription only.** 800-232-5512 http://www.mpmmedicalinc.com
Remedy Repair Crème	Medline Industries Inc.	Helps restore natural moisture balance to skin while delivering vital nutrients. Moisturizes/protects skin.	Pharmacies. 800-633-5463 http://www.medline.com
Siberian Seabuckthorn oil	Survivor input	Promotes healing of heat burns, radiation burns, sunburns, poorly healing wounds, bedsores, skin ulcers, eczema.	Online stores. http://www.floraleads.com

continues

Products for Radiation Dermatitis *continued*

Product	Source	Description	How to Access
Spand-Gel™ Wound Dressing	Medi-Tech International Corp.	Provides moist, cool wound-healing environment. Relieves pain, burning, itching, and soreness. Contains aloe vera. Available as a neck wrap.	800-333-0109 http://www.medi-techintl.com http://www.balegoonline.com http://www.amazon.com
Udderly Smooth® Hand & Foot Cream	Redex Industries Inc.	Used to treat dry skin. Contains urea to enhance moisturizing. Smoothes roughness and softens skin. Unscented.	800-345-7339 http://www.udderlysmooth.com http://www.drugstore.com
Vigilon® Gel Dressings	C.R.Bard Medical	Cools/reduces pain of skin tears, minor burns, and radiation reactions. Absorbent, nonadherent hydrogel dressing. Natural anesthetic effect.	800-397-5899 http://www.vitalitymedical.com 800-861-3211 http://www. http://AllegroMedical.com
Vitamin E capsules and aloe vera gel	Patient input	Pierce a vitamin E capsule and apply contents to skin every night; remove before radiation treatments. Apply aloe vera on skin directly after treatment.	**Consult your radiation oncologist.** Pharmacies. Vitamin shops.
Xclair™ Cream	Align Pharmaceuticals	Increases hydration, reduces inflammation & soothes the skin damaged by radiation therapy. Does not contain steroids, immunomodulating substances, alcohol, or fragrance.	**Consult your physician. By prescription only.** 908-834-0960 http://www.align.com

Products and Therapies to Help Reduce the Side Effects of Neck Dissections

Product	Source	Description	How to Access
Acupuncture	Survivor input	Used for the treatment of pain in the neck and shoulders resulting from neck dissection surgery.	**Consult your physician.**
Barnes Myofascial Release	Survivor input	Hands-on technique that provides sustained pressure into connective tissue to relieve pain and restore motion from tightness and restriction to the fascia caused by physical trauma, scarring, stress, and inflammation.	**Consult your physician.** **Consult a physical therapist.** http://www.myofascial release.com
Botox® (botulinum toxin)	Allergan Inc.	Used to help stop muscle spasms. Injection.	**Consult your physician.** **By prescription only.**
Celebrex® (celecoxib)	Pfizer	Used to relieve pain, tenderness, swelling, and stiffness.	**Consult your physician.** **By prescription only.** 800-438-1985
Physical therapy	Survivor input	For deep tissue release of muscle spasms and contracture of muscles.	**Consult your physician.** **Consult a physical therapist.**

continues

Products and Therapies to Help Reduce the Side Effects of Neck Dissections *continued*

Product	Source	Description	How to Access
Soma® (carisoprodol)	MedPoint Pharmaceuticals	Relaxes muscles and relieves pain and discomfort. A muscle relaxant, used with rest, physical therapy, etc. May cause drowsiness.	**Consult your physician. By prescription only.**
Trigger point massage therapy	Survivor input	Applies concentrated pressure to areas of chronic or severe pain in the muscles, called "trigger points." May help to free frozen shoulder.	**Consult your physician. Consult a physical therapist.**

Products to Help Relieve Lhermitte's Sign

(Electriclike shocks extending down the spine upon flexing the head caused by radiation toxicity to the central or peripheral nervous system)

and

Neuropathy

(Numbness, tingling sensation, muscle weakness, pain in the extremities)

Product	Source	Description	How to Access
Acupuncture	Survivor input	May help to reduce pain.	**Consult your physician.** 510-649-8488 http://www.hmieducation.com

Product	Source	Description	How to Access
Elavil® (amitriptyline)	Merck	Sometimes used to treat chronic pain. Also used in the treatment of Lhermitte's sign at low doses. Considered a tricyclic antidepressant.	**Consult your physician. By prescription only.**
Lidoderm® (lidocaine patch)	Endo Pharmaceuticals Inc.	Used to relieve pain. Class of medications called local anesthetics. Works by stopping nerves from sending pain signals.	**Consult your physician. By prescription only.**
Neurontin® (gabapentin)	Pfizer	May help to relieve the pain of neuropathy and Lhermitte's sign at low doses. Class of medications called anticonvulsants. Tablet or liquid form.	**Consult your physician. By prescription only.** 800-438-1985
Tegreto® (carbamazepine)	Novartis Pharmaceuticals	Used in the treatment of Lhermitte's sign at low doses. Tablet or liquid form. Anticonvulsant.	**Consult your physician. By prescription only.**
Tofranil® (imipramine)	Mallickrodt Inc.	Used in the treatment of Lhermitte's sign at low doses. A tricyclic antidepressant. Tablet.	**Consult your physician. By prescription only.**
Transcutaneous electrical nerve stimulation (TENS)	TENS units made by different manufacturers	Works to decrease pain perception and may be used to control acute and chronic pain. Battery-operated stimulator.	**Consult your physician. Consult a physical therapist.** Online stores.

173

Products to Help Relieve Pain

Product	Source	Description	How to Access
Acupuncture	Patient input	May help to reduce pain. Specific areas of the body are shallowly pierced with fine needles to relieve pain or produce regional anesthesia.	**Consult your physician.** 510-649-8488 http://www.hmieducation.com
Duragesic® (fentanyl topical)	Janssen Pharmaceutical Products LP	Used to relieve pain. A narcotic (opioid) pain medicine. May cause drowsiness.	**Consult your physician. By prescription only.** 800-526-7736
Liquid Motrin® (ibuprofen)	McNeil Consumer Healthcare	Used to help relieve pain. Easier to swallow than tablet.	Pharmacies. Supermarkets. 877 223-9807
Liquid Tylenol®	McNeil Consumer Healthcare	Used to help relieve pain. Easier to swallow than tablet.	Pharmacies. Supermarkets. 877 223-9807
OxyContin® (oxycodone)	Purdue Pharma	Used to relieve moderate to severe pain. May cause drowsiness. Liquid and tablet form.	**Consult your physician. By prescription only.** 888-726-7535
Prialt® (ziconotide)	Elan Pharmaceuticals	Used to treat severe chronic pain. May cause drowsiness.	**Consult your physician. By prescription only.** 800-859-8586.
Therapeutic nerve blocks	Survivor input	Used to control pain. Nerve blocks contain local anesthetic. Injection.	**Consult your physician. By prescription only.**

174

Products and Therapies to Help Reduce Lymphedema

Product/Therapy	Description	How to Access
Compression bandaging	Used to treat lymphedema. Compression options may be difficult with facial edema. Bandaging with short stretch bandages and sometimes combined with various types of foam. May help break up fibrosis (thickening) in tissues as well as reduce the volume of edema.	**Consult your physician.** **Consult a physical therapist.** National Lymphedema Network http://www.lymphnet.org
Compression garments	Can be custom made to wear during sleeping or for periods of time to add compression in the face.	**Consult your physician.** **Consult a physical therapist.** National Lymphedema Network http://www.lymphnet.org
Eucerin® or Curél®	Use to provide good skin care and hygiene to help avoid infections and wounds.	Pharmacies. Supermarkets. 800-227-4703
Exercise	Used to improve biomechanical function and soften the tissues under the skin of the face and neck to reduce swelling. "Facial gymnastic exercises," deep breathing exercises. Pool exercise is excellent for lymphedema.	**Consult your physician.** **Consult a physical therapist.** National Lymphedema Network http://www.lymphnet.org
Lymphedema alert bracelets	Used to provide awareness of lymphedema. Bracelets say: "Lymphedema Alert: No blood pressure and no needles into this arm."	National Lymphedema Network http://www.lymphnet.org
MLD (manual lymph drainage)	Designed to shift the lymphatic fluid from congested areas to normal ones.	**Consult your physician.** **Consult a physical therapist.**

Products to Treat Anemia Caused by Poor Nutrition

Products	Description	How to Access
Cobalamin (vitamin B_{12})	Used in the treatment of pernicious anemia and anemia resulting from a lack of vitamin B_{12}. Given by injection.	**Consult your physician.** Pharmacies. Online stores
Folic acid (B-complex vitamin)	Used for the treatment of folic acid deficiency anemia resulting from low levels of folic acid in the body caused by poor nutrition, poor absorbtion, and some medications.	**Consult your physician.** Pharmacies, health food stores.
Oral iron supplements (ferrous sulfate)	Used for iron deficiency anemia caused by too little iron in the diet, poor absorption of iron by the body, and gastrointestinal blood loss caused by ulcers and the use of aspirin and nonsteroidal anti-inflammatory medications (NSAIDS). Liquid prescriptions may stain teeth.	**Consult your physician.** Pharmacies, health food stores.

Products to Help With Chemotherapy-Induced Anemia

Product	Source	Description	How to Access
Aranesp® (darbepoetin alfa)	Amgen	May be given as a series of injections to induce bone marrow to make more red blood cells.	**Consult your physician. By prescription only.**
Epogen® (epoetin alfa)	Amgen	May be given as a series of injections to induce bone marrow to make more red blood cells.	**Consult your physician. By prescription only.**
Procrit® (epoetin alfa)	Ortho Biotech Inc.	May be given as a series of injections to induce bone marrow to make more red blood cells.	**Consult your physician. By prescription only.**

Products to Help With Fatigue*

Product	Source	Description	How to Access
Carnitor® (levocarnitine)	Sigma-Tau Pharmaceuticals Patient input	Used to treat fatigue resulting from carnitine deficiency caused by chemotherapy or poor nutrition. Injection, capsules, or liquid.	**Consult your physician. By prescription only.**
Provigil® (modafinil)	Cephalon	Improves wakefulness. May promote a sense of well-being, decreased fatigue, and increased appetite. Psychostimulant for cancer patients.	**Consult your physician. By prescription only.**
Ritalin® (methylphenidate hydrochloride)	Novartis Pharmaceuticals	May help cancer patients fight fatigue (otherwise used to treat attention deficit hyperactivity disorder in children).	**Consult your physician. By prescription only.**
Synthroid® (levothyroxine)	Abbott Laboratories	May help to decrease fatigue associated with reduced thyroid function.	**Consult your physician. By prescription only.**

*Treating anemia may also help fatigue.

Products to Help With Dehydration

Product	Source	Description	How to Access
Bouillon and broths	Many manufacturers	Provides hydration and electrolytes.	Supermarkets. Convenience stores. Online stores.
Gatorade®	Gatorade Company	Provides essential hydration, salt replacement, and energy boost.	Pharmacies. Supermarkets. Online stores.
Pedialyte®	Abbott Laboratories	Provides a balance of fluid and proper electrolytes to restore proper hydration.	Pharmacies. Supermarkets. Convenience stores. Online stores.
Sports drinks: Powerade Accelerade Lucozade Sport	Many manufacturers	Helps to rehydrate and replenish electrolytes, sugar, water, and other nutrients.	Pharmacies. Supermarkets. Convenience stores. Online stores.
ZIP-N-SQUEEZE®	ZNS Products	Encourages hydration: A squeezable product to help with hydration and liquid nutrition. No sucking required. For use when cups and straws are difficult or cannot be used. For patient care following head and neck cancer rehabilitation (swallowing must be intact).	714-997-7146 http://www.zip-n-squeeze.com

Products to Help With Nausea

Product	Source	Description	How to Access
Acupuncture	Survivor input	May help in the treatment of nausea.	**Consult your physician.** 510-649-8488 http://www.hmieducation.com
Compazine® (prochlorperazine)	GlaxoSmithKline (GSK)	Used to treat nausea/vomiting. Tablet, extended release capsule, oral liquid, rectal suppository. May cause drowsiness.	**Consult your physician. By prescription only.** 888-825-5249
Zofran®	GlaxoSmithKline (GSK)	Used to prevent nausea and vomiting that may be caused by chemotherapy, radiation therapy, and surgery. Tablet and liquid.	**Consult your physician. By prescription only.** 888-825-5249

Products to Help Relieve Constipation

Product	Source	Description	How to Access
Aloe vera juice	Survivor input	Drink 3 to 4 mouthfuls at a time to help relieve constipation.	Health food stores.
Colace®	Purdue Pharma LP	Indicated for the treatment of occasional constipation. Capsules, liquid, suppositories.	Pharmacies. Supermarkets. Online drugstores. 800-877-5666
Dose of medication	Survivor input	Use of some medications may cause constipation. Dose may need to be adjusted.	**Consult your physician.**
Dulcolax® (bisacodyl)	Boehringer Ingelheim Consumer Healthcare	Used on a short-term basis to treat constipation. Tablet, suppository.	Pharmacies. Supermarkets.
A home remedy for bowel regularity	Survivor input	Mix ⅔ cup oat bran, ⅔ cup prune juice, and ⅔ cup unsweetened applesauce. Eat a few tablespoons to ½ cup, twice daily. Refrigerate unused portion for later use.	Supermarkets for ingredients.
Metamucil® (Psyllium)	Procter & Gamble	Contains psyllium husk, a natural dietary fiber that relieves constipation and can lower blood cholesterol levels. Powder, granules, and wafer.	Pharmacies. Supermarkets. Online drugstores.

Product	Source	Description	How to Access
Miralax®	Schering-Plough Healthcare Products	Used to treat occasional constipation. Powder laxative, Mixed with a liquid and taken by mouth	**Consult your physician. Prescription only.** http://www.drugstore.com
Senakot®	Purdue Pharma L.P.	Works by irritating bowel tissues resulting in bowel movements. Stimulant laxative. Tablet.	Pharmacies. Supermarkets. Online drugstores.
Smooth Move® herbal stimulant laxative tea	Traditional Medicinals Survivor input	Provides gentle and effective overnight relief. A sweet-tasting citrus-flavored herbal tea. Chocolate flavor also available.	Supermarkets. Whole Foods. Trader Joe's. Vitamin World. http://www.traditional medicinals.com http://www.drugstore.com

Products to Help Relieve Diarrhea

Product	Source	Description	How to Access
Imodium® AD (loperamide)	McNeil Consumer Healthcare	Used to control diarrhea. Tablet, capsule, and liquid to take by mouth.	Pharmacies. Supermarkets. Online stores.
Kaopectate®	Chattem Inc.	Used to treat mild to moderate diarrhea. Tablet, chewable tablet, liquid. Take by mouth.	Pharmacies. Supermarkets. Online stores.
Lomotil® (diphenoxylate with atropine)	Pfizer	Used to control diarrhea. Works by slowing the movement of the intestines. Tablet and liquid forms.	**Consult your physician. By prescription only.** 800-438-1985
Sandostatin® (octreotide)	Novartis Pharmaceuticals	Helps control diarrhea and other symptoms of abdominal illness. Injection	**Consult your physician. By prescription only.**

Additional Side Effects of Treatment

Description	How to Access
Ear Pain and Hearing Loss	
Radiation may cause swelling and obstruction of the eustachian tubes causing fluid to collect in the middle ear and/or swelling of the external ear canal. Usually temporary condition. Ventilation tubes may be necessary to relieve negative pressure when condition persists.	Consult your physician.
Fluid in the ear following head and neck surgery may occur following surgery on the maxillary sinus and palate. Usually temporary condition. Ventilation tubes may be necessary to relieve negative pressure when condition persists.	Consult your physician.
Ear pain may be caused by hardening of the wax in the ear.	Consult your physician.
Ear pain may be caused by persistent tumor of the throat.	Consult your physician.
Loss of Smell and Taste	
Loss of taste may occur as a result of mucositis and radiation effects on the taste buds (papillae). As papillae regenerate, sense of taste may return, usually after a few months.	Consult your radiation oncologist.
Loss of smell may be, in part, due to the loss of taste. Usually returns upon return of taste. Consult your radiation oncologist.	Consult your radiation oncologist.
Dry Eyes	
Dry eyes may result from irradiation of the lacrimal (tear-producing) glands, which are located in the upper outer part of the eye sockets. They may be affected during treatment for cancers close to or involving the eyes or sinuses. Use of tear substitutes should be used to prevent dry eyes and further complications.	Consult your ophthalmologist.

Treating Toxicities From Targeted Therapies

Products to Help Treat Skin Rash

(Skin rash is a common side effect of treatment using targeted therapies.)

Product	Source	Description	How to Access
Accutane® (isotretinoin)	Roche Pharmaceuticals and others	Used to treat severe acne that has not been helped by other treatments. Oral medication.	**Consult your physician. By prescription only.**
Aclovate® (alclometasone dipropionate)	GlaxoSmithKline Pharmaceuticals	Used to treat skin problems that are accompanied by itching, redness, and swelling. Synthetic corticosteroid. Cream, ointment.	**Consult your physician. By prescription only.** 800-645-9833
Atarax® (hydroxyzine)	Pfizer	Use to relieve severe itching. Also used to relieve anxiety and tension. Has sedative effect.	**Consult your physician. By prescription only.** 800-438-1985
Bactroban® Ointment (mupirocin)	GlaxoSmithKline (GSK)	Used to treat impetigo as well as other skin infections caused by bacteria.	**Consult your physician. By prescription only.** 888-825-5249
Cipro® (ciprofloxacin)	Bayer Pharmaceuticals	Used to treat infections caused by bacteria. An antibiotic. Tablet and suspension.	**Consult your physician. By prescription only.** 888-842-2937

Product	Source	Description	How to Access
Doryx® (doxycxcyline)	Warner Chilcott Laboratories	Prevents the growth and spread of bacteria. Antibiotic taken by mouth to reduce inflammations of the skin. Pill or liquid form.	**Consult your physician. By prescription only.**
Dynacin® (minocyline)	Medicis Pharmaceuticals Corp.	Used to treat bacterial infections, acne, and infections of the skin. A tetracycline antibiotic.	**Consult your physician. By prescription only.** 602-808-8800
Elidel® (pimecrolimus 1% cream)	Novartis Pharmaceuticals	Shown to control the redness, inflammation, and itching of eczema. A topical cream.	**Consult your physician. By prescription only.** 800-277-2254
Metrogel® (metronidazole gel, topical)	Galderma Laboratories LP	Used in the topical treatment of inflammatory lesions of the skin.	**Consult your physician. By prescription only.** 866-735-4137
Regenecare® Wound Gel	MPM Medical Inc.	Used to reduce rash and itching caused by EGFR drugs. A pain-relieving hydrogel. Contains lidocaine HCl, collagen, and aloe vera.	**Consult your physician. By prescription only.** 800-232-5512 http://www.mpmmedicalinc.com

continues

Products to Help Treat Skin Rash *continued*

Product	Source	Description	How to Access
Regenecare® HA Wound Gel	MPM Medical Inc.	Used to treat skin problems such as itching and rash associated with EGFR drugs. Contains lidocaine HCl, collagen, aloe vera, and hyaluronic acid (HA).	**Consult your physician. By prescription only.** 800-232-5512 http://www.mpmmedicalinc.com 800-461-1370 http://www.suprememedical.com
Sumycin® (tetracycline)	Par Pharmaceuticals Inc.	Used to reduce inflammations of the skin. Prevents growth and spread of bacteria. An antibiotic. Capsule and liquid.	**Consult your physician. By prescription only.** 800-828-9393
Terramycin® (tetracycline)	Pfizer	Prevents the growth and spread of bacteria. Antibiotic taken by mouth to reduce inflammations of the skin. Pill or liquid form.	**Consult your physician. By prescription only.** 800-438-1985

Products to Help Relieve Itchy Dry Skin and Dry Nails

Product	Source	Description	How to Access
Aveeno® Soothing Bath Treatment	Johnson & Johnson	Used for temporary relief of itchy, dry, sensitive skin. Fragrance free with colloidal oatmeal.	Pharmacies. Supermarkets. Online drug stores.
Allegra®	Sanofi-Aventis	Used for relief of dry itchy skin. An Antihistamine. May cause dry mouth. May cause drowsiness.	**Consult your physician. By prescription only.**
Baking soda baths	Survivor input	1 to 2 cups baking soda in lukewarm bath water. May help to reduce itchy skin.	Supermarkets for ingredients.
Benadryl®	McNeil Consumer Healthcare	Used for relief of dry itchy skin. An Antihistamine. May cause dry mouth. May cause drowsiness.	Pharmacies. Supermarkets. Online drug stores.
Carmol®10	Doak Dermatologics	Used to help restore and retain normal skin softness. Total body lotion for dry skin. 10% urea.	Pharmacies. Online drug stores
Claritin®	Schering-Plough Health Care Products	Used for relief of dry, itchy skin. May cause dry mouth and drowsiness.	Pharmacies. Supermarkets. Online drug stores

continues

187

Products to Help Relieve Itchy Dry Skin and Dry Nails *continued*

Product	Source	Description	How to Access
Clobex® (clobetasol)	Galderma Laboratories, L.P.	Used for treatment of itchy, redness, dryness, crusting, scaling, inflammation, and discomfort of skin and scalp conditions. May also help relieve inflammation of nail areas. Cream or ointment.	**Consult your physician. By prescription only.** 866-735-4137
Cormax® (clobetasol)	Oclassen Pharmaceuticals Inc.	Used to treat itchy, redness, dryness, crusting, scaling, inflammation, and discomfort of skin and scalp conditions. May also help to relieve inflammation of nail areas. Cream or ointment.	**Consult your physician. By prescription only.**
Dermablend® concealment makeup	Dermablend	Does not contain fragrance or alcohol. Dermatologist tested, Allergy tested, Will not clog pores. Will not cause acne.	http://www.dermablend.com
Kenalog® (triamcinolone)	Bristol-Myers Squibb Company	Used to treat the itching, redness, dryness, crusting, scaling, inflammation, and discomfort of various skin conditions. Helps reduce skin infections around the nails. A synthetic corticosteroid.	**Consult your physician. By prescription only.**
Lidex® (fluocinonide)	Medicis Pharmaceuticals Corp.	Used to treat the itching, redness, dryness, crusting, scaling, inflammation, and discomfort of various skin conditions. A synthetic corticosteroid cream.	**Consult your physician. By prescription only.**

Product	Source	Description	How to Access
Lindi® Face Serum	Lindi Skin Products	Used to hydrate the face, neck, shoulders, and upper body	800-380-4704 http://www.lindiskin.net Use online retail store locator.
Lindi® Face Wash	Lindi Skin Products	Used to moisturize irritated and sensitive skin. Good for those with sensitivity to soap.	800-380-4704 http://www.lindiskin.net Use online retail store locator.
Lindi® Lip Balm	Lindi Skin Products	Used to help with dry or cracked lips. May also help hydrate nail beds and cuticles.	800-380-4704 http://www.lindiskin.net Use online retail store locator.
Loprox® (ciclopirox)	Medicis Pharmaceuticals Corp.	Used in the treatment of fungal and yeast infections of the skin. Topical cream, gel, or lotion.	**Consult your physician.** **By prescription only.**
Lyrica® (Pregabalin)	Pfizer	Helps to control severe symptoms of itching.	**Consult your physician.** **By prescription only.** 800-438-1985
New-Skin® Antiseptic Liquid Bandage	Medtech Labs Inc.	Apply to nail areas at first sign of skin cracking to prevent inflammation. Keeps out moisture, allowing the skin to heal.	Pharmacies. Supermarkets. Online drugstores.
Sarna Ultra® Anti-Itch Cream	Stiefel Laboratories Inc.	Used to relieve itching associated with dry, rough, cracked skin.	Pharmacies. Online drugstores. 888-784-3335

continues

Products to Help Relieve Itchy Dry Skin and Dry Nails *continued*

Product	Source	Description	How to Access
Temovate® (clobetasol propionate cream)	PharmaDerm	Used to treat itchiness, redness, dryness, crusting, scaling, inflammation, discomfort of various skin and scalp conditions. A synthetic corticosteroid. May also help to relieve inflammation of nail areas.	**Consult your physician. By prescription only.**
Vinegar soaks	Home remedy	Helps to decrease nail disease and lowers risk of infection and spread of bacteria. Mix 1 part white vinegar with 10 parts water. Soak affected fingers or toes several times a day for 5 minutes or more.	Supermarket for ingredients.
Vistaril® (hydroxyzine)	Pfizer	Used to relieve itchy skin. An antihistamine. Capsules, tablets, a syrup, and suspension.	**Consult your physician. By prescription only.** 800-438-1985
Westcort® (hydrocortisone valerate steroid cream)	Bristol-Myers Squibb Company	Helps to relieve itching redness and swelling caused by a wide variety of skin conditions, such as acne-like rash. A synthetic (man-made) corticosteroid.	**Consult your physician. By prescription only.**

Products to Help Moisturize and Heal Dry Skin and Nails

Product	Source	Description	How to Access
Aquaphor® Healing Ointment	Eucerin	Protects dry, cracked or irritated skin to help enhance the natural healing process and restore smooth, healthy skin.	Pharmacies. Supermarkets. Online drugstores. 800-227-4703 http://www.eucerinus.com
Aveeno® Moisturizing Bar	Johnson & Johnson Consumer Products Companies	Moisturizes and cleanses dry, sensitive skin. Soap free, hypoallergenic. Formulated with natural oatmeal.	Pharmacies. Supermarkets. Online drugstores. 800-526-3967
Basis® Sensitive Skin Bar Soap	Beiersdorf	Cleans dry, sensitive skin with almond oil, chamomile, and aloe vera.	Pharmacies. Supermarkets. Online drugstores. 800-233-2340
Cetaphil® Antibacterial Gentle Cleansing Bar	Galderma Laboratories, L.P	May be used to treat inflamed areas of the skin surrounding nails. Antibacterial soap for dry, sensitive skin.	Pharmacies. Supermarkets. Online drugstores. 866-735-4137
Cetaphil® Gentle Cleansing Bar	Galderma Laboratories, L.P	Helps restore moisture and is a gentle, nonalkaline, nonsoap cleanser for dry, sensitive skin.	Pharmacies. Supermarkets. Online drugstores. 866-735-4137
Cetaphil® Moisturizing Lotion	Galderma Laboratories, L.P	Helps restore skin's natural protective barrier. Fragrance free, non-comedogenic, non-greasy. Moisturizes skin and reduce itch.	Pharmacies. Supermarkets. Online drugstores. 866-735-4137

continues

Products to Help Moisturize and Heal Dry Skin and Nails *continued*

Product	Source	Description	How to Access
Desenex®	Novartis Consumer Health	Used in the treatment of superficial fungal infections of the skin. Relieves itching, burning and irritation. Antibiotic, anti-fungal powder, cream, spray.	Pharmacies. Supermarkets. Online drugstores. 800-277-2254
Dove® Sensitive Skin Unscented Beauty Bar	Unilever	Moisturizes dry and sensitive skin. Helps to reduce itch. Fragrance-free hypoallergenic.	Pharmacies. Supermarkets. Online drugstores.
Eucerin® Original	Eucerin	Heals and protects very dry sensitive skin. Fragrance-free, non-comedogenic, non-irritating. Lotion and Cream.	Pharmacies. Supermarkets. Online drugstores. 800-227-4703 http://www.eucerinus.com
Lotrimin® (clotrimozole)	Schering-Plough Health Care Products	Used to prevent nail areas from becoming infected. Antifungal ointment, cream, spray, powder.	Pharmacies. Supermarkets. Online drugstores. 800-222-7579
Neutrogena® Facial Cleansing Bar	Neutrogena Corp.	Glycerine-rich bar that contains no harsh detergents, dyes, or hardeners. Dry skin, fragrance-free formula available.	Pharmacies. Supermarkets. Online drugstores. 800-582-4048
Neutrogena® Norwegian Formula Hand Cream	Neutrogena Corp.	Helps heal dry, chapped hands. Concentrated, glycerine-rich formula.	Pharmacies. Supermarkets. Online drugstores. 800-582-4048

192

Product	Source	Description	How to Access
Neutrogena® Ultra Sheer™ Dry-Touch Sunblock SPF 55 with Helioplex™	Neutrogena Corp.	Offers protection for sensitive skin. Broad-spectrum UVA/UVB. PABA free. Helioplex™ helps prevent damaging UVA rays from penetrating deep under skin's surface.	Pharmacies. Supermarkets. Online drugstores.
Vanicream® Cleansing Bar	Pharmaceutical Specialties Inc.	Moisturizes while gently cleansing skin. Free of fragrance and common chemical irritants.	Pharmacies. 800-325-8232 http://www.psico.com
Vanicream® Lite Lotion	Pharmaceutical Specialties Inc.	Moisturizes and soothes red, dry, irritated, cracking, or itchy skin.	Pharmacies. 800-325-8232 http://www.psico.com
Vanicream® moisturizing skin cream	Pharmaceutical Specialties Inc.	Moisturizes and soothes red, irritated, cracking, or itchy skin.	Pharmacies. 800-325-8232 http://www.psico.com
Vanicream® sunscreen	Pharmaceutical Specialties Inc.	Protects skin from the sun without the use of sensitizing chemical sunscreens. Effectively blocks both UVA and UVB. Free of preservatives, dyes, perfume, lanolin, formaldehyde, PABA and benzophenones. 30, 35 and 60 SPF.	Pharmacies. 800-325-8232 http://www.psico.com
Vaseline® Intensive Care Advanced Healing Lotion	Unilever	Hydrates & heals extra dry skin. Leaves skin feeling silky smooth and comfortable. Fragrance free.	Pharmacies. Supermarkets. Online drugstores.

continues

Products to Help Moisturize and Heal Dry Skin and Nails *continued*

Product	Source	Description	How to Access
Vaseline® Petroleum Jelly	Unilever	Apply a thick coat of Vaseline to hands and feet at night; cover with white cotton gloves and socks. Helps to moisturize and keep nails and skin from drying out.	Pharmacies. Supermarkets. Online drugstores. 800-272-6296

Alternative/Complementary Treatments That Survivors Have Found Helpful

Product	Source	Description	How to Access
Chinese herbal medicine	Survivor input	Refers to herbs used in combinations for many conditions. May be used to reduce pain, stiffness, fatigue, and inflammation.	**Consult your physician.** http://www.nccam.nih.gov
Massage	Survivor input	Refers to an assortment of techniques involving manipulation of the soft tissues of the body through pressure and movement.	**Consult your physician.** http://www.nccam.nih.gov

Product	Source	Description	How to Access
Meditation	Survivor input	Refers to a group of meditation techniques used for various health problems, including anxiety, pain depression, mood and self-esteem problems, stress, insomnia, and physical or emotional symptoms that may be associated with chronic illnesses and their treatment.	**Consult your physician.** http://www.nccam.nih.gov
Qigong	Survivor input	Refers to an energy modality involving the coordination of different breathing patterns with various physical postures and motions of the body to help improve health through the reduction of stress and exercise.	**Consult your physician.** http://www.nccam.nih.gov
Reflexology	Survivor input	Refers to a method of foot and hand massage in which pressure is applied to "reflex" zones of the feet and hands to help improve general health.	**Consult your physician.** http://www.nccam.nih.gov

continues

Alternative/Complementary Treatments That Survivors Have Found Helpful *continued*

Product	Source	Description	How to Access
Reiki	Survivor input	Refers to a healing energy that is channeled through a practitioner's hands. May induce relaxation; improve immunity; and reduce pain, stress, anxiety, and depression.	**Consult your physician.** http://www.nccam.nih.gov
Tai chi	Survivor input	Refers to moving the body slowly and gently, while breathing deeply and meditating. Used to improve physical condition, muscle strength, coordination, and flexibility. Also used to ease pain and stiffness.	**Consult your physician.** http://www.nccam.nih.gov
Yoga	Survivor input	Refers to a mind-body medicine typically focusing on intervention strategies that are thought to promote health and well-being.	**Consult your physician.** http://www.nccam.nih.gov

Appendix

PROGRAMS OF OUTREACH AND SUPPORT, LITERATURE, WEB SITES, AND ORGANIZATIONS

Support for People with Oral and Head and Neck Cancer (SPOHNC), a patient-directed self-help organization, was founded in 1991 by an oral cancer survivor. This nonprofit organization is dedicated to raising awareness and meeting the emotional, physical, and humanistic needs of oral and head and neck cancer patients and their families and friends.

SPOHNC offers two programs of outreach and support for patients with oral and head and neck cancer. Its National Survivor Volunteer Network (NSVN) is a network of more than 125 survivor volunteers who communicate on a one-to-one basis with newly diagnosed patients or recovering patients. Patients may phone 800-377-0928 or e-mail info@spohnc.org to be matched with a volunteer who can provide information, support, and encouragement to those in need.

Chapters of SPOHNC are found throughout the United States. These chapters hold monthly meetings offering information, support, and encouragement to newly diagnosed patients, survivors, family members, and friends in a friendly and nonthreatening forum. Survivors share their situations, experiences, coping strategies, and hopes. Educational presentations by health care professionals are also part of the SPOHNC program. Some chapters are facilitated by health care professionals, and others are facilitated by cancer survivors. SPOHNC chapters strive to provide survivors a support system tailored to their individual needs.

Following is a list of SPOHNC chapters. In some cities, there is more than one chapter. A complete listing of chapters and contact information can be found on SPOHNC's Web site at http://www.spohnc.org. Additional information about specific chapters can also be obtained by calling SPOHNC's office at 800-377-0928.

Arizona—Phoenix

Arizona—Scottsdale

Arkansas—Northwest

California—Los Angeles

California—Orange County

California—Paso Robles

California—San Diego

California—Stanford

Colorado—Denver

Florida—Boca Raton

Florida—Englewood

Florida—Fort Walton Beach

Florida—Gainesville

Florida—Lecanto

Florida—Miami

Florida—Ocala

Florida—Orlando

Florida—Sarasota

Georgia—Atlanta

Illinois—Chicago

Illinois—Maywood

Indiana—Indianapolis

Kansas—Kansas City

Louisiana—Baton Rouge

Maryland—Baltimore

Massachusetts—Boston

Massachusetts—Peabody

Michigan—Detroit

Michigan—Troy

Minnesota—Minneapolis

Missouri—St. Louis

Montana—Bozeman

North Carolina—Charlotte

Nebraska—Omaha

New Jersey—Long Branch

New Jersey—Morristown

New Jersey—Philadelphia

New Jersey—Toms River

New Mexico—Albuquerque

New York—Albany

New York—Buffalo

New York—Manhattan

New York—Rochester

New York—Stony Brook

New York—Syosset

New York—Westchester

Ohio—Cleveland

Ohio—Columbus

Ohio—Kettering

Oklahoma—Tulsa

Oregon—Medford

Pennsylvania—Mechanicsburg

Pennsylvania—Monroeville

Texas—Dallas

Texas—Fort Worth

Texas—Houston/Tomball

Virginia—Charlottesville

Virginia—Fairfax

Virginia—Norfolk

Washington, DC

Wisconsin—Madison

Literature, Web Sites, and Organizations Sources of Information for Coping With Oral and Head and Neck Cancer

Books About Oral and Head and Neck Cancer

Clarke, L. K., & Dropkin, M. J. (2006). *Head and neck cancer.* Pittsburgh, PA: Oncology Nursing Society.

Clifford, K. S. C., & Ozyigit, G. (Eds.). (2003). *Intensity modulated radiation therapy.* Philadelphia, PA: Lippincott Williams & Wilkins.

Harrison, L. B., Sessions, R. B., & Hong, W. K. (2004). *Head and neck cancer, a multidisciplinary approach.* Philadelphia: Lippincott Williams & Wilkins.

Lydiatt, W., & Johnson, P. (2001). *Cancers of the mouth and throat, a patient's guide.* Omaha, NE: Addicus Books.

Shah, J. P. (Ed.). (2001). *Cancer of the head and neck*, a volume in the American Cancer Society *Atlas of Clinical Oncology* series. Hamilton, Ontario, Canada: BC Decker.

SPOHNC (Support for People with Oral and Head and Neck Cancer). (2006). *Eat well—Stay nourished, a recipe and resource guide for coping with eating challenges.* Lenexa, KS: Cookbook Publishers.

SPOHNC. (2006). *We have walked in your shoes.* Locust Valley, NY: Author.

Wang, C. C. (1996). *Radiation therapy for head and neck neoplasms.* New York: Wiley-Liss.

Autobiographies

Cohen, H. (2006). *Risen from the ashes—Tales of a musical messenger.* Lanham, MD: Hamilton Books.

Fleming, T. (1999). *A rendezvous with Clouds.* Albuquerque, NM: University of New Mexico Press.

Grealy, L. (1994). *Autobiography of a face.* New York: HarperCollins.

Healey, T. (2006). *At face value—My triumph over a disfiguring cancer.* Ashland, OR: Caveat Press.

Phelan, W. A. (2006). *Running with cancer: The ultimate marathon.* Bloomington, IN: AuthorHouse.

Cancer Web Sites for Oral and Head and Neck Cancer

Adenoid Cystic Carcinoma Organization International
P.O. Box 15482
San Diego, CA 92175
http://www.accoi.org

Adenoid Cystic Carcinoma Research Foundation
P.O. Box 442
Needham, MA 02494
http://www.accrf.org

American Academy of Otolaryngology-Head and Neck Surgery (AAO-HNS)
One Prince Street
Alexandria, VA 22314
703-836-4444
http://www.entnet.org

American Head & Neck Society
11300 W. Olympic Boulevard, Suite 600
Los Angeles, CA 90064
310-437-0559
http://www.ahns.info

International Association of Laryngectomees (IAL)
P.O. Box 12036
Jacksonville, NC 28546
910-340-4519
http://www.larynxlink.com

National Cancer Institute (NCI)
Public Inquiries Office
Building 31, Room 10A31
31 Center Drive, MSC 2580, Bethesda, MD 20892
800-4-CANCER (800-422-6237)
http://www.cancer.gov

National Institute of Dental and Craniofacial Research (NIDCR)
Bethesda, MD 20892
301-402-7364
http://www.nidcr.nih.gov

National Organization for Rare Disorders (NORD)
55 Kenosia Avenue
P.O. Box 1968
Danbury, CT 06813-1968
203-744-0100; 800-999-6673 (voice mail only)
http://www.rarediseases.org

The Oral Cancer Foundation
3419 Via Lido #205
Newport Beach, CA 92663
949-646-8000
http://www.orlcancerfoundation.org

Society of Otorhinolaryngology and Head-Neck Nurses (SOHN)
116 Canal Street, Suite A
New Smyrna Beach, FL 32168
386-428-1695
http://www.sohnnurse.com

Support for People with Oral and Head and Neck Cancer (SPOHNC)
P.O. Box 53, Locust Valley, NY 11560
800-377-0928
http://www.spohnc.org

WebWhispers
Terry Duga
6115 North Park Avenue
Indianapolis, In 46220
http://www.webwhispers.org

The Yul Brynner Head and Neck Cancer Foundation
P.O. Box 250550
Charleston, SC 29425
843-792-0546
http://www.headandneck.org

General Cancer Books and Magazines

Anderson, G., & Simonton, C. (1999). *Cancer: 50 essential things to do*. New York: Plume.

Armstrong, L. (2001). *It's not about the bike: My journey back to life*. New York: Berkley Trade.

Canfield, J. (1996). *Chicken soup for the soul: 101 healing stories about those who have survived cancer*. Deerfield, FL: HCI.

Coping With Cancer magazine, P.O. Box 682268, Franklin, TN 37068-2268; 615-790-2400; http://www.coping.com

CURE magazine, 3535 Worth Street, Collins Tower, Suite 185, Dallas, TX 75246; 800-210-CURE; http://www.curetoday.com

Fincannon, J. L., & Bruss, K. V. (2003). *Couples confronting cancer: Keeping your relationship strong*. Atlanta, GA: American Cancer Society.

Geffen, J. (2000). *The Journey through cancer*. New York: Crown.

Granet, R. (2001). *Surviving cancer emotionally: Learning how to heal*. New York: John Wiley & Sons.

Groopman, J. (2004). *The anatomy of hope*. New York: Random House.

Heal—Living Well After Cancer magazine, 3500 Maple Avenue, Suite 750, Dallas, TX 75219; 800-210-2873; http://www.healtoday.com

Hermann, J. F. (2001). *Cancer in the family: Helping children cope with a parent's illness*. Atlanta, GA: American Cancer Society.

Hoffman, B. (1996). *A cancer survivor's almanac: Charting your journey*. Minneapolis, MN: Chronimed.

Holland, J. C., & Lewis, S. (2001). *The human side of cancer: Living with hope, coping with uncertainty*. New York: Harper.

Kushner, H. S. (2004). *When bad things happen to good people*. New York: Anchor.

Schlessel Harpham, W. (2003). *Diagnosis: Cancer* (Exp. Ed.). New York: W. W. Norton.

Schlessel Harpham, W. (2005). *Happiness in a storm*. New York: W. W. Norton.

Zakarian, B. (1996). *Activist cancer patient: How to take charge of your treatment*. New York: John Wiley & Sons.

Organizations

American Association for Cancer Research
615 Chestnut Street, 17th Floor
Philadelphia, PA 19106
215-440-9300/866-423-3695
http://www.aacr.org

American Cancer Society
1599 Clifton Road, NE
Atlanta, GA 30329
800-227-2345
http://www.cancer.org

American Dental Association (ADA)
211 East Chicago Avenue
Chicago, IL 60611
312-440-2500
http://www.ada.org

American Dietetic Association
120 South Riverside Plaza, Suite 2000
Chicago, IL 60606-6995
800-877-1600
http://www.eatright.org

American Institute for Cancer Research
1759 R Street, NW
Washington, DC 20009
800-843-8114
http://www.aicr.org

American Psychosocial Oncology Society
2365 Hunters Way
Charlottesville, VA 22911
434-293-5350
http://www.apos-society.org

American Society of Clinical Oncology (ASCO)
1900 Duke Street, Suite 200
Alexandria, VA 22314
703-299-0150
http://www.asco.org

American Society for Therapeutic Radiology & Oncology (ASTRO)
8280 Willow Oaks Corporate Drive, Suite 500
Fairfax, VA 22031
800-962-7876

703-502-1550
http://www.astro.org

Cancer Care
275 Seventh Avenue
New York, NY 10001
800-813-HOPE (800-813-4673)
212-712-8400
http://www.cancercare.org/

Corporate Angel Network Inc. (CAN)
Westchester County Airport
One Loop Road
White Plains, NY 10604
866-328-1313
914-328-1313
http://www.corpangelnetwork.org

Department of Veteran Affairs
800-827-1000
http://www.va.gov

Fertile Hope
65 Broadway
New York, NY 10006
888-994-4673
http://www.fertilehope.org

Gilda's Club Worldwide
322 Eighth Avenue, Suite 1402
New York, NY 10001
888-445-3248
917-305-1200
http://www.gildasclub.org

Lance Armstrong Foundation
P.O. Box 161150
Austin, TX 78716
877-236-8820
512-236-8820
http://www.laf.org

Look Good...Feel Better
c/o CTFA Foundation
1101 17th Street, NW
Washington, DC 20036
202-331-1770
http://www.lookgoodfeelbetter.org

MedlinePlus—Trusted Health Information for You
A Service of the U.S. National Library of Medicine and the
National Institutes of Health
8600 Rockville Pike
Bethesda, MD 20894
http://www.medlineplus.gov

National Association for Home Care
228 Seventh Street, SE
Washington, DC 20003
202-547-7424
http://www.nahc.org

National Association of Social Workers
750 First Street, NE, Suite 700
Washington, DC 20002
800-638-8799
http://www.socialworkers.org

National Cancer Institute's Cancer Information Service (CIS)
6116 Executive Boulevard, Room 3036A
Bethesda, MD 20892
800-4-cancer (800-422-6237)
cis.nci.nih.gov

National Comprehensive Cancer Network
500 Old York Road, Suite 250
Jenkintown, PA 19046
888-909-NCCN
215-690-0300
http://http://www.nccn.org

National Family Caregivers Association
10400 Connecticut Avenue, Suite 508
Kensington, MD 20895
800-896-3650
301-942-6430
http://www.nfcacares.org

National Library of Medicine
8600 Rockville Place
Bethesda, MD 20894
888-346-3656
301-594-5983
http://www.nlm.nih.gov

National Organization for Rare Disorders (NORD)
55 Kenosia Avenue
P.O. Box 1968
Danbury, CT 06813
203-744-0100
http://www.rarediseases.org

NeedyMeds
120 Western Avenue
Gloucester, MA 01930
http://www.needymeds.com

People Living With Cancer
1900 Duke Street, Suite 200
Alexandria, VA 22314
888-651-3038
http://www.plwc.org

Planet Cancer
314 E. Highland Mall Boulevard, Suite 260-17
Austin, TX 78752
512-452-9010
http://www.planetcancer.org

R.A. Bloch Cancer Foundation
4400 Main Street
Kansas City, MO 64111
800-433-0464
816-932-8453
http://www.blochcancer.org

RadiologyInfo
820 Jorie Boulevard
Oak Brook, IL 60523
630-571-2670
http://www.radiologyinfo.org

Surveillance Epidemiology and End Results (SEER)
National Cancer Institute
Suite 504, MSC 8316
6116 Executive Boulevard
Bethesda, MD 20892-8316
http://www.seer.cancer.gov

The Wellness Community
919 18th Street, NW, Suite 54
Washington, DC 20006
888-793-WELL (888-793-9355)
202-659-9709
http://www.thewellnesscommunity.org

INDEX